D1635956

The Board's Role in Quality Care

A Practical Guide for Hospital Trustees

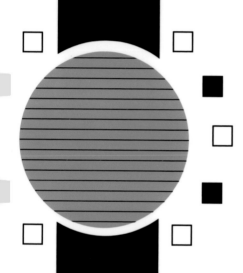

James E. Orlikoff
and Mary K. Totten

AHA

The Board's Role in Quality Care

A Practical Guide for Hospital Trustees

WITHDRAWN

James E. Orlikoff and Mary K. Totten

AHA

AHA books are published by
American Hospital Publishing, Inc.,
an American Hospital Association company

The views expressed in this publication are strictly those of the authors and do not necessarily represent official positions of the American Hospital Association.

Library of Congress Cataloging-in-Publication Data

Orlikoff, James E.
    The board's role in quality care : a practical guide for
hospital trustees / James E. Orlikoff and Mary K. Totten.
        p.   cm.
    ISBN 1-55648-061-X
    1. Hospital care–Quality control.
    2. Hospitals–Trustees. I. Totten, Mary K. II. Title.
    [DNLM: 1. Governing Board. 2. Hospital Administration.
    3. Quality Assurance, Health Care.   WX 150 071b]
    RA972.O753   1991
    362.1'1'0685–dc20
    DNLM/DLC
    for Library of Congress   90-14512
                                                              CIP

Catalog no. 196126

©1991 by American Hospital Publishing, Inc.,
an American Hospital Association company

Printed in the USA

AHA is a service mark of the American Hospital Association used under license by American Hospital Publishing, Inc.

Text set in Palatino
4.5M—02/91—0289
4M—09/92—0332

Richard Hill, Project Editor
Linda Conheady, Manuscript Editor
Sophie Yarborough, Editorial Assistant
Marcia Bottoms, Managing Editor
Peggy DuMais, Production Coordinator
Marcia Vecchione and Susan Edge-Gumbel, Designers
Brian Schenk, Books Division Director

Contents

About the Authors iv

List of Figures and Table v

Chapter 1. Introduction 1

Chapter 2. A Brief History of the Concern for Quality 5

Chapter 3. Why Hospital Boards Are Responsible
for Quality 21

Chapter 4. Becoming Comfortable with the Basics
of Quality 35

Chapter 5. Effectively Overseeing Quality
and Quality Assurance 55

Chapter 6. The Board's Role in Medical Staff Credentialing 73

Chapter 7. Improving the Board's Information
about Quality 91

Chapter 8. Quality and Board Organizational Structure 115

Chapter 9. New Approaches in Quality:
Continuous Quality Improvement 129

Chapter 10. Conclusion 149

About the Authors

James E. Orlikoff is president of Orlikoff & Associates, a Chicago-based consulting firm specializing in health care leadership, quality, and risk management. He was formerly the director of the American Hospital Association's Division of Hospital Governance and the director of the Institute on Quality of Care and Patterns of Practice of the AHA's Hospital Research and Educational Trust.

Mr. Orlikoff has been involved in quality, leadership, and risk management issues for over 10 years. He has designed and implemented hospital quality assurance and risk management programs in four countries, and since 1985 has worked with hospital governing boards to strengthen their overall effectiveness and their oversight of quality assurance and medical staff credentialing. He has written five books and over 40 articles and currently serves on hospital and civic boards.

Among Mr. Orlikoff's publications are *Malpractice Prevention and Liability Control for Hospitals* (1988), *Quality from the Top: Working with Hospital Governing Boards to Assure Quality Care* (1990), and *The Guide to Governance for Hospital Trustees* (1990).

Mary K. Totten is president of Totten & Associates, an Oak Park, IL, consulting firm specializing in health care leadership. She was formerly the program director for the Division of Hospital Governance of the American Hospital Association.

Ms. Totten has been a speaker and consultant to over 40 hospital boards and hospital associations on quality of care, medical staff credentialing, liability exposure, and governance issues. She has managed grant projects and published monographs, briefing papers, and articles for hospital trustees on quality issues. She has worked with national trustee leaders to assess the governing board's responsibility for quality care and has developed discussion forums and publications on defining and measuring quality for health care purchasers and providers.

Among Ms. Totten's publications are *The Guide to Governance for Hospital Trustees* (1990).

List of Figures and Table

Figures

Figure 2-1. Legal Relationships among the Governing Body, Administration, and Medical Staff (pre-1965) 18

Figure 2-2. Legal Relationships among the Governing Body, Administration, and Medical Staff (current) 19

Figure 4-1. Internal and External Perspectives of Quality 39

Figure 6-1. Examples of Level 2 Medical Staff Quality-Related Credentialing Criteria 87

Figure 6-2. Sample Level 1 and Level 2 Evaluation Form 88

Figure 7-1. Possible Indicators of Quality for the Board, by Internal and External Category and by Perspective of Quality 103

Figure 7-2. Sample Board Quality Indicator Report: Graph of Hospitalwide Nosocomial Infections 108

Figure 7-3. Sample Board Quality Indicator Report: Graph of Hospitalwide Nosocomial Infections, with Addition of Threshold Line 109

Figure 7-4. Sample Board Quality Indicator Report: Graph of Hospitalwide Mortalities as a Percentage of Discharges, with an Inappropriate Threshold Line 110

Figure 7-5. Sample Board Quality Indicator Report: Graph of Hospitalwide Mortalities as a Percentage of Discharges, with a More Appropriate Threshold Line 111

Figure 7-6. Sample Board Report: Incident Reports by Category,
1/1/90 to 12/31/91.................................112

Figure 7-7. Sample Board Report: Incident Reports Compared
to Malpractice Claims, 1/1/90 to 12/31/91.............113

Figure 8-1. Sample Role Statement of the Board
Quality Committee................................120

Figure 8-2. Sample Organizational Chart for a Board
with a Quality Committee.........................121

Figure 8-3. Sample Organizational Chart for a Board Quality
Committee That Does Not Review Medical Staff QA
or Credentials Information and Recommendations....122

Figure 9-1. Deming's 14 Points for Continuous
Quality Improvement.............................136

Figure 9-2. The Seven Deadly Diseases Inhibiting
Quality Improvement.............................137

Figure 9-3. Common Scientific Tools and Their Uses
for Continuous Quality Improvement...............139

Figure 9-4. Sample Pareto Chart for Identifying Opportunities
for Quality Improvement.........................139

Figure 9-5. Sample Cause-and-Effect Diagram for Identifying
Opportunities for Quality Improvement.............140

Figure 9-6. Quality Project Milestones.........................142

Table

Table 3-1. Hospitals with the Highest and Lowest 1987
Mortality Rates for Coronary-Artery Bypass
Surgery on Medicare Patients.....................31

Chapter 1

Introduction

Does your hospital deliver high-quality care to its patients? If you are like most hospital trustees, you would answer yes to that question. Now consider this question: How do you *know* that your hospital provides high-quality care?

Most trustees answer that question in one of the following three ways. "I know that my hospital provides good care because: 1. We are accredited by the Joint Commission on Accreditation of Healthcare Organizations." Or, "2. because we have a quality assurance program and it generates so many reports I can't help but believe that it must be doing something to improve the quality of care." Or, "3. because we have a Board quality assurance committee, a joint conference committee, a hospitalwide quality assurance committee, and a medical staff quality assurance committee."

These common responses indicate that most hospital governing board members sincerely want to believe that their hospital delivers quality care. When they seriously examine the question, however, they find that they really do not know much about the quality of care in their hospital at all. For example, ask yourself these questions. Is my hospital's quality of care better or worse than it was last year? Better or worse than last quarter? What are my hospital's strengths in quality? What are the weaknesses? How has the board positively influenced the hospital's quality of care in the past year? If you can recall reasonably *specific* answers to those questions, then you are in a minority of hospital trustees who are both meaningfully aware of their hospitals' quality of care, and whose boards probably take an active role in improving their hospitals' quality of care.

If you cannot reasonably answer those questions, then you have a lot in common with the majority of hospital trustees and boards. Unfortunately, most hospital boards are unclear as to what their responsibility is for the quality of care in their hospitals. Further, most trustees and boards are unaware of what the various levels of quality are in their hospitals. Most important, the majority of hospital boards do not know how to effectively and appropriately oversee quality assurance programs and quality improvement activities in their hospitals to meaningfully improve the quality of care.

Pressures are mounting for boards to accept, clarify, and actively discharge their responsibility for assuring and improving their hospital's quality of care. These pressures come from many sources, including the federal government, the courts, regulatory and accrediting agencies, the media, third-party payers of hospital services, the public, and many others. These pressures for quality are growing and will increasingly have an impact on hospitals and, more specifically, on the boards that govern them.

Why should your hospital board be actively concerned with its hospital's quality of care? Although that question will be addressed in depth throughout this book, it is worth touching on here. Basically, quality of care is becoming a strategic imperative for hospitals. In other words, hospitals are rapidly entering the era when they will *compete* on the basis of the quality of care and service that they provide.

During the 1980s hospitals, pressured by the federal government's revamped financing system (the prospective payment system, or PPS), were compelled by new hospital market forces to learn how to compete on cost and price. Those hospitals that learned to control costs within the prospective payment system survived, and some even prospered. Those hospitals unable to compete within the environment of constrained costs closed, merged, or otherwise radically changed.

In any maturing market, the natural progression is movement from competition on *cost and price* to competition on *quality*. This evolution of competition from cost to quality is classically seen in tightening markets. As the health care market tightens and becomes increasingly efficient and unforgiving, hospitals will be forced to compete on quality as well as on cost and price. This growing trend can already be seen in the public release of comparative indicators of hospital quality, such as the Medicare mortality data that are released annually by the federal government.

Furthermore, the important relationship between cost and quality will in itself force increasing scrutiny and control of the quality of care by hospitals and their boards. To remain competitive, hospitals must actively seek ways of providing the highest-quality care at the lowest possible cost. At the same time, the regulatory, accrediting, and hospital licensing agencies are stepping up their efforts to require that hospitals demonstrate they are in fact providing high-quality care. Those hospitals that cannot do so risk serious sanctions, loss of licensure, and closure.

Therefore, for many reasons, a board must be concerned with the quality of care provided by its hospital. The very survival of the hospital in the future will depend in large part on the quality of care it provides. As hospitals increasingly compete on quality, those that do so effectively will survive and prosper; those that do not will go out of business.

Thus hospital boards will find that quality of care is an issue they are spending more time, energy, and resources on. Hospitals that survive and thrive in the coming tumultuous years will do so largely because they have organized to effectively assess and continuously improve their quality of care. For hospitals to sincerely and effectively manage for quality, hospital boards must sincerely and effectively govern for quality.

Unfortunately, significant barriers currently preclude many boards from effectively governing for quality. One barrier is that many trustees are intimidated by the concept that they bear responsibility for quality of care within their institutions. Further, many trustees are intimidated by the very notion of quality of care. "After all," many trustees think, "don't you have to be a physician to understand quality?" The corollary to that thinking is often expressed by many trustees: "Isn't quality the job of the medical staff?"

In addressing those questions and many more, this book is intended help you feel comfortable with the issues of quality, quality assurance, total quality management and continuous quality improvement, medical staff credentialing, risk management, and related activities. This book will demonstrate *why* the board has the ultimate responsibility for quality and will clarify the role of the board regarding quality and medical staff credentialing. It will then present understandable strategies and techniques to help you and your board effectively discharge the board's crucial responsibility for quality.

There is a noble and worthwhile purpose to these activities: to deliver the best quality of care possible and to strive always to improve that care. Thus true quality is best regarded as a goal or journey as opposed to an attainable end.

Consequently, the organizational commitment to quality is the foundation that supports all quality assurance and quality improvement activities. Although the structures and mechanisms of the quality assurance program and medical staff activities are key in expressing this commitment to quality, it is ultimately the organization's commitment to quality that engenders a true quest for and continuous improvement of quality. The commitment to the quality journey must spring from, and be renewed and supported by, the board.

Think of this book as your guide to your board's and hospital's quest for quality. It will not always be an easy journey, and there are certain to be adventures and surprises. It is, however, a journey that must be approached with passion by an organization. That passion for quality, for the quest for quality, must come from the top of the organization, that is, from the board. Are you ready to begin the journey?

Chapter 2

A Brief History of the Concern for Quality

Introduction

Because the issue of quality of care is raised with increasing frequency in today's health care environment, it is easy to assume that the concern for quality in health care is a relatively recent development. Although the emphasis on quality is indeed stronger than ever before, the concern for quality in health care is in fact almost as old as the practice of medicine itself.

To help provide you with an important perspective on this issue, this chapter will briefly trace the evolution of the concern for quality and quality assurance in medicine and hospitals. It will also stress the evolution of the responsibility for quality and present the background necessary to understand why the hospital board now bears the ultimate responsibility for the quality of care and for the quality assurance program and related activities of the hospital.

The Code of Hammurabi

About 2000 B.C. in Babylonia there lived an emperor named Hammurabi. Hammurabi has the dubious distinction of being generally considered the father of modern bureaucracy, for it was he who institutionalized the practice of writing extensive laws that governed Babylonian society, including their professional and commercial activities and enterprises.

Hammurabi wrote the very first law that addressed the issues of quality of care, malpractice, and accountability and liability for the provision of substandard care. As quoted in Kramer (1976), the Code of Hammurabi stated:

If the surgeon has made a deep incision in the body of a free man
and has caused the man's death or has opened the caruncle in the
eye and so destroys the man's eye, they shall cut off his forehand.

From this starting point at about 2000 B.C., most subsequent societies in some way sanctioned the practice of medicine. But it is with
Hammurabi in ancient Babylonia that the origin of society's concern
for quality care is found.

Even though the Code of Hammurabi is almost 4,000 years old and
sprang from another culture, there are several points worth noting in
Hammurabi's law that have a direct bearing on how the issue of quality is practically and conceptually regarded in the United States today.
First, notice that Hammurabi's law addresses the issue of malpractice
and of avenues available for patients to redress their grievances against
physicians. Yet the law also addresses the issue of the quality of patient
care. Thus the concern for quality of care grew from, or at least strongly
related to, the concern for malpractice prevention and compensation—or
retribution—for malpractice.

The notion that the issue of quality relates to the issue of malpractice began with Hammurabi's law and in fact persists to this day. Just
as in Hammurabi's time, many of the concerns for quality hospital care
in the United States relate directly to issues of malpractice and malpractice liability for substandard care. In fact, as will be discussed later in
this chapter, much of the current emphasis on quality—as well as the
hospital board's responsibility for quality and oversight of the medical
staff—developed as a direct result of medical malpractice cases.

Another significant point evident in Hammurabi's law is the implicit
definition of quality. Notice that Hammurabi's law defines quality care
not by what it *is* but, rather by what it *is not*. In other words, quality
is defined not as a *positive characteristic* of care but as the *absence of negative characteristics*. In Hammurabi's law, quality is implicitly defined as
not causing a free man's death or as *not* destroying a man's eye. These
negative characteristics or outcomes of care can be described by the term
disquality. Thus the definition of quality in Hammurabi's law is the
absence of disquality. This is in fact the primary way quality care is con-
ceptualized and measured today, not by what is positive in care but rather
by the absence of disquality. This points out the difficulty, apparent even
4,000 years ago, in both defining and measuring the quality of care. The
issue, still critically important today, can be clarified in this paraphrase
of a famous statement: "I don't know what quality of care is, but I know
it when I *don't* see it."

Still another point in Hammurabi's law, perhaps the most important, is the issue of who is held accountable for the quality, or disquality, of care. Notice that the law holds the individual physician to be the

ultimate responsible and accountable authority for the quality or disquality of care provided to patients. The hospital or hospital board was not held responsible primarily because there were no hospitals or boards as such in ancient Babylonia.

The notion that responsibility and accountability for quality of care rest ultimately with the individual physician persisted for thousands of years; only recently did this notion expand to hospitals and their boards. The evolutionary process for responsibility for quality went something like this:

1. Individual physicians had the ultimate authority and responsibility.
2. Organized physicians (the medical staff) within the hospital had the ultimate authority and responsibility.
3. As a corporate institution the hospital had authority and responsibility.
4. The hospital board had ultimate authority and responsibility.

Understanding this evolution and expansion of the responsibility for quality is critical to understanding many issues relating to the board's role in quality and the quality of care in hospitals. The issues include:

- Why the board has ultimate responsibility and accountability for quality
- Why the medical staff often resists and resents the board's responsibility
- Why trustees are often uncomfortable with this responsibility
- Why it is often a difficult responsibility for boards to effectively discharge.

All of these points will be addressed in depth throughout this book.

It is critical to note that the issue of quality of care inexorably intertwines with the issue of *who is responsible* for the quality of that care. Hammurabi's law specified that it was the individual physician who ultimately had the responsibility and accountability for quality. This notion persisted for thousands of years, and, in the minds of many physicians, trustees, managers, and patients, it persists to this day.

Evolution and expansion of ultimate responsibility for quality from the physician to the medical staff to the hospital to the board is a critical issue in the assurance and continuous improvement of the quality of care in hospitals and health care organizations. A critical and delicate issue that remains from this evolution is clarification of the relative roles and responsibilities of the physician, the medical staff, management, and the governing board regarding quality care.

Clearly, as a trustee or as a patient, you would want your physician to have a strong sense of responsibility for the quality of care he or she provides. Further, you would want the medical staff to have a strong sense of responsibility and accountability for monitoring and improving the quality care provided by your physician. Finally, you might recognize that the hospital and its governing board also share responsibility and accountability for the quality of care provided by the individual physician. The tricky issue is: What is the difference in these responsibilities and how can all involved hospital groups reconcile and accept these different but related responsibilities? This extremely important issue has its roots in the brief but significant Code of Hammurabi.

One other side issue can also be seen in Hammurabi's law. Notice that the law relates only to quality of care and avenues of retribution for "a free man." Did quality of care or malpractice prevention not apply to slaves and women? Thus in Hammurabi's law it is also possible to see the origins of an institutionalized two-tiered system of health care. Today it is said there is one health care system for people with money and/or health insurance coverage and another system of poorer-quality health care for those without money or health insurance. The two-tiered system is often discussed as an unfortunate component of the current health care system in the United States.

It can be argued, then, that the brief law of Hammurabi contains the roots of many significant issues related to quality of care in hospitals today. These critical issues include the relationship of quality to malpractice, how quality is defined and measured, who is ultimately responsible and accountable for the quality of care, and who should have access to high-quality care.

The Hippocratic Oath

About 1,600 years after the Code of Hammurabi, a Greek physician named Hippocrates advanced a school of medicine that stressed diet, medicinal waters, fresh air, and physical fitness. One of the characteristics of Hippocrates's school of medicine was the requirement that those young men about to enter the field of medicine take an oath.

This oath that Hippocrates was said to require of his disciples related to physician adherence to a code of medical ethics. The Hippocratic Oath, dated to about 400 B.C., contained the phrase *primum non nocere,* which in Latin roughly translates to the concept that the physician should "first do no harm." In this simple phrase can be seen several concepts that reflect Hammurabi's perspective on quality and that still influence our own to this day.

First, just as Hammurabi's did, Hippocrates' approach to defining quality care rested on the *absence of disquality.* Further, the oath implies that quality care is present when harm or injury to the patient has been prevented. The phrase "first do no harm" clearly states that one of the first duties of the physician is to not cause injury to the patient.

Second, once again it is the individual physician who is held to be the ultimate responsible authority regarding the quality of patient care. This was true because the relationship of the physician to the patient was seen by Hippocrates as being a helping and healing one between two people. The intensely interpersonal nature of the physician–patient relationship was, in ancient Greece, unencumbered by technological procedures or organizational structures such as hospitals or medical staffs. Thus, it was the individual physician, adhering to his admirable code of medical ethics, who was the final responsible authority for the quality of care provided.

Hippocrates, often regarded as the father of medicine, further advanced the notion that the individual physician carried the ultimate responsibility for the quality of care because Hippocrates ended the tradition of the priest–physician. In separating the physician from the priest he removed the notion that God retained ultimate responsibility for outcome and quality of care and advanced the notion that this responsibility rested with the individual physician.

The Work of Florence Nightingale

Several thousand years subsequent to Hammurabi and Hippocrates, the concept that the individual physician bore ultimate responsibility for the quality of care rendered to the patient took root and blossomed. Even though the 18th century saw the advent of hospitals, the hospital as such was not regarded as having responsibility for quality; that was the domain of the physician.

Perhaps the first individual to challenge this concept was Florence Nightingale, an English philanthropist, naturalist, nurse, and student of hospital management. In 1854, during the Crimean War, Nightingale headed a group of nurses in a British barrack-hospital, tending to the wounded of the battlefields (Cohen, 1984).

Nightingale introduced many innovative measures to the care of the patients; these included sanitation, ventilation, drainage, the use of disinfectants, and diet, among others. Because of her efforts, the mortality rate among patients in the barrack-hospital declined dramatically.

Nightingale developed several concepts that directly relate to the hospital's responsibility for, and techniques for achieving, standards of quality. She clearly demonstrated that the hospital as an organization could positively and dramatically influence the quality of care provided to patients.

She also pioneered a technique still used in hospital quality assurance programs today, that of the retrospective review of care. Nightingale saw that the military patients could be grouped according to their wounds or diseases. She reasoned that not all groups of patients would benefit equally from the medical resources that the barrack-hospital had to offer. So she conducted a retrospective review of patients treated by the hospital to determine which past groups of patients benefited the most from treatment, and thus which future groups of patients should be given the highest priority for treatment. Thus she originated the concept of *triage,* that the sickest patients who would benefit from treatment be treated first (rather than first come, first served), which is still used in U. S. emergency departments. To conduct this process of retrospective review, Nightingale gathered mortality and morbidity data to identify patterns of care and then used this information to improve the care that would be provided to future patients.

As a result of these innovative activities Nightingale developed two powerful concepts in quality. The first was that the hospital as an organization could influence and improve the quality of care it provided. The second was that by examining the quality of care the hospital had provided to patients in the past, the hospital could identify ways of providing better-quality care to patients in the future. Both concepts were extremely powerful and would exert tremendous influence on the development of the concern and responsibility for quality of care in hospitals.

Early Concerns for Quality of Care in America

From the founding of the first hospital in the United States in 1752 by Benjamin Franklin (who was the first American hospital trustee) to the mid-1950s, responsibility for quality rested primarily, if not completely, with the individual physician or with groups of physicians. The hospital as an organization, as well as the board as the ultimate authority of the organization, had no real responsibility for the quality of care.

This attitude toward high physician responsibility and low or nonexistent board responsibility can be seen in the 1902 Michigan Supreme Court ruling in *Pepke v. Grace,* where the board of a Michigan hospital believed it should be more active in overseeing the activities of the medical staff via more rigorous board involvement in the medical staff credentialing process. The medical staff disagreed with the board and in fact took umbrage at the board's temerity in questioning the authority of the physician as ultimate authority for quality. The medical staff sued the board, and the case went to the Michigan Supreme Court, which ruled:

> The trustees of a hospital are laymen. The rules of the hospital provide for a medical board . . . , who have charge of all surgical matters

in the hospital. They examine applicants . . . , and recommend such appointments to the trustees. . . . The trustees, who are laymen, must naturally leave the competency of the physician . . . to the judgment of those competent to determine such matters, since they are not qualified to make the determinations themselves. (The board) performed their full duty . . . in appointing a (medical) board to examine applicants.

The *Pepke v. Grace* ruling reinforced the prevalent and, unfortunately, still-persistent perspective that the board's role in deciding which physicians could be members of the medical staff, and which clinical privileges they could or could not have, was little more than that of a rubber stamp. The board was expected, and in fact was required by the Michigan Supreme Court, to simply approve without review or question all recommendations from the medical staff credentials or executive committee. This approach to board responsibility, or more precisely *lack of responsibility*, included the issue of the quality of care in addition to oversight of the medical staff.

In 1914, 12 years after *Pepke v. Grace*, a court ruling in the state of New York clearly emphasized the hospital governing board's, and the hospital organization's, complete lack of responsibility for the quality of medical care provided by the hospital. In *Schloendorff v. Society of New York Hospital*, the New York State Court of Appeals held that hospitals were responsible only for the ministerial care or administrative acts of their employees. The court also ruled that hospitals, or the governing boards of hospitals, were not responsible for the medical care provided by physicians or nurses or other health care providers. Nurses and other health care providers were regarded by the court as subject to the direction of the physician, not the hospital.

Around the time of the *Schloendorff* ruling an American physician named Ernest Amory Codman read Florence Nightingale's book, *Notes on Nursing*, which described her innovations and their positive effects on the quality of care provided to the wounded soldiers fighting for England in the Crimean War. Codman reasoned that those same innovations and techniques applied in American hospitals would result in better quality of care. So, around 1915 Codman went to the medical staff of his hospital and urged them to evaluate the end results of their care and act on the results of that evaluation to improve the quality of care.

Unfortunately, the medical staff was not impressed with Codman's idea. After all, was not the individual physician responsible for providing quality care, and thus for looking after his own care? Had this not been the case for thousands of years? The medical staff was so infuriated by

Codman's suggestions and heretical ravings that they quickly ejected him from membership in the medical staff.

Codman was not dissuaded from his mission of improving the quality of care. He continued to urge medical professionals to evaluate and improve the quality of their care and to become accountable to the public, instead of simply to themselves.

In 1916 Codman published a book, *A Study in Hospital Efficiency,* in which he outlined his theories and called on hospitals and the medical profession to embrace them. Codman stated in his book:

> I am called eccentric for saying in public that hospitals, if they wish to be sure of improvement:
> - Must find out what their results are;
> - Must analyze their results to find their strong and weak points;
> - Must compare their results with those of other hospitals;
> - Must care for what cases they can care for well, and avoid attempting to care for cases which they are not qualified to care for well;
> - Must assign the cases to members of the staff (for treatment) for better reasons than seniority, the calendar, or temporary convenience;
> - Must welcome publicity not only for their successes, but for their errors, so that the public may give them their help when it is needed;
> - Must promote members of the staff on the basis which gives due consideration to what they can and do accomplish for their patients.
>
> Such opinions will not be eccentric a few years hence.

Codman was clearly a man ahead of his time, for in this statement can be seen many of the same quality-related issues being frequently discussed, debated, and emphasized today. Those issues include the release of quality data that facilitate comparisons about quality between and among hospitals, the notion that not all hospitals should offer all types of medical services, the concept of the hospital's responsibility to oversee the medical staff by the use of credentialing systems, the notion of the accountability of hospitals to the public, and many others.

Perhaps the most important characteristic in the concepts advanced by Codman was that the organized medical staff, as well as the hospital as an organization, carried a responsibility for the quality of care that transcended that of the individual physician. Thus after thousands of years the concept that ultimate authority and responsibility for quality rested on the individual physician, as advanced by Hammurabi and Hippocrates, was being challenged.

The Expansion of Responsibility for Quality of Care

Although Codman was not much heeded by the medical staff at his own hospital, he did influence the medical profession. In 1917, one year after Codman's book was published, the American College of Surgeons published a "Minimum Standard" that was designed to instill some standardization of practice among American hospitals and recognize hospitals devoted to providing high-quality care to patients. This Minimum Standard was the basis for the American College of Surgeons' Hospital Standardization Program, the first accreditation program for hospitals in the United States. In part, as quoted in the American College of Surgeons (1924), the Minimum Standard stated:

1. That physicians and surgeons privileged to practice in the hospital be organized as a definite group or staff. . . .
2. That membership upon the staff be restricted to physicians and surgeons who are (a) full graduates of medicine in good standing and legally licensed to practice in their respective states or provinces, (b) competent in their respective fields, and (c) worthy in character and in matters of professional ethics; that in this latter connection the practice of the division of fees, under any guise whatever, be prohibited.
3. That the staff initiate and, with the approval of the governing board of the hospital, adopt rules, regulations, and policies governing the professional work of the hospital; that these rules, regulations, and policies specifically provide:
   (a) That staff meetings be held at least once each month. . . .
   (b) That the staff review and analyze at regular intervals their clinical experience in the various departments of the hospital . . . ; the clinical records of patients, free and pay, to be the basis for such review and analyses.
4. That accurate and complete records be written for all patients and filed in a manner accessible to the hospital. . . .
5. That diagnostic and therapeutic facilities under competent supervision be available for the study, diagnosis, and treatment of patients. . . .

In 1918, the American College of Surgeons initiated a voluntary hospital accreditation program based on compliance with the Minimum Standard. Thus the Minimum Standard constituted the first explicit requirements that related to the responsibility of the *hospital* to monitor and evaluate the quality of patient care (Joint Commission on Accreditation of Healthcare Organizations, 1988, p. 11).

Even though the Minimum Standard was the first to address the hospital's responsibility for quality, it is important to point out that that responsibility was largely a ceremonial one; the lion's share of the burden and the responsibility for the review of quality was placed with the medical staff, not with the hospital as an organization. In fact, the only reference to the responsibility of the hospital is seen in standard #3 that "the approval of the governing board of the hospital" is given to the medical staff's "rules, regulations, and policies" that relate to the review and assurance of quality.

It is easy to get the sense from the Minimum Standard that the role of the board, and thus the hospital as an organization, was primarily that of a rubber stamp regarding quality and oversight of the medical staff. That a medical organization such as the American College of Surgeons would be interested in the notion of minimizing a lay board's authority over the medical staff is not surprising. Thus the Minimum Standard perpetuated the perspectives seen in the *Pepke v. Grace* and *Schloendorff* rulings, that the responsibility of the hospital and its board for quality was at most minimal and pro forma.

Nevertheless, the Minimum Standard and the Hospital Standardization Program (which was the name of the first hospital accreditation program in the United States) of the American College of Surgeons are quite significant in the evolution of the concern for quality of care in the United States. The Minimum Standard represents the beginning of the expansion of the responsibility for quality from the individual physician to an organized *group* of physicians: the hospital medical staff. Thus, 4,000 years of historical imperative for the responsibility for quality that began with Hammurabi were beginning to change.

The Joint Commission on Accreditation of Hospitals

From the inception of the Minimum Standard, the idea grew that the medical staff was primarily responsible for quality, with a cursory nod from the governing board. Over time, more hospitals voluntarily applied to the American College of Surgeons' Hospital Standardization Program to be surveyed to see whether they complied with the Minimum Standard. If they did, they received a stamp of approval, accreditation, from the Hospital Standardization Program.

In 1918, the first year of the Hospital Standardization Program, 89 hospitals received approval, and by 1951 that number had grown to more than 3,000 (Joint Commission on Accreditation of Healthcare Organizations, 1988, p. 11). It was determined that an independent organization solely devoted to expanding and improving voluntary hospital accreditation was needed. Thus in 1951 the American College of Surgeons, the American College of Physicians, the American Medical Association, the

American Hospital Association, and the Canadian Medical Association established the Joint Commission on Accreditation of Hospitals (Joint Commission). The Canadian Medical Association withdrew from sponsorship in 1959 and was replaced in 1979 by the American Dental Association.

In 1953 the Joint Commission published the *Standards for Hospital Accreditation*, which was an expanded and updated version of the Minimum Standard. The *Standards* contained brief guidelines on hospital bylaws, buildings, governing bodies, dietary services, food preparation, and nursing services. The *Standards* specified that the medical staff conduct quality-related review activities and report results to the medical staff executive committee (Joint Commission on Accreditation of Healthcare Organizations, 1988, p. 11).

The Joint Commission did not yet have standards that specifically addressed the hospital's responsibility to conduct quality assurance or quality review activities. Further, the *Standards* did not recognize, address, or specify the board's responsibility for quality, other than another requirement that the board give "rubber stamp" approval to the recommendations of the medical staff. The initial standards of the Joint Commission were, again, minimal standards for quality.

The Growing Responsibility of the Hospital

As can be seen in the previous two sections, the development in the concern for quality of care in hospitals from 1918 to 1953 focused primarily on the responsibilities and activities of the organized medical staff. Thus the expansion of the ultimate authority and responsibility for quality from the individual physician to the organized medical staff continued and solidified.

In the late 1950s, however, a series of malpractice cases began to change the environment for quality responsibility even more. These cases began to define the *hospital's* responsibilities for quality and for medical staff oversight and in the process expanded the hospital's liability for failing to effectively discharge that responsibility. (So, once again the influence of Hammurabi—the linkage of the concern for quality to the issue of malpractice—is evident.) These cases signaled the beginning of the increasing responsibilities of the hospital and its board for quality.

Bing v. Thunig

Perhaps the first malpractice case that marked this next step in the evolution and expansion of responsibility for quality was *Bing v. Thunig* in New York in 1957. The following quotation from the ruling of the New

York Court of Appeals clearly demonstrates the expansion of the responsibility for quality beyond the individual physician or organized medical staff to include the hospital as an organization:

> The conception that the hospital does not undertake to treat the patient, does not undertake to act through its doctors and nurses, but undertakes instead simply to procure them to act upon their own responsibility, no longer reflects the fact. Present day hospitals . . . do far more than furnish facilities for treatment. They regularly employ on a salary basis a large staff of physicians, nurses, and interns, . . . and they charge patients for medical care and treatment, collecting for such services, if necessary, by legal action. Certainly, the person who avails himself of "hospital facilities" expects that the hospital will attempt to cure him, not that its nurses or other employees will act on their own responsibility. Hospitals should, in short, shoulder the responsibilities borne by everybody else.

Thus hospitals were now regarded as having some responsibility for the quality of care they provided. It was only a matter of time before this responsibility expanded further to include the ultimate authority of the hospital—its governing board.

Darling v. Charleston Community Memorial Hospital

In 1964 in Charleston, Illinois, a young man named Darling suffered a fractured right leg during a football game. He was taken to Charleston Community Memorial Hospital's emergency room, where he was seen by the physician on call. That physician, Dr. Alexander, performed an orthopedic treatment to the boy's leg, applied a cast to the leg, and admitted him to the hospital as his patient. It was later noted that Dr. Alexander was not experienced in orthopedic work of this nature.

During Darling's stay in the hospital he complained of pain in his leg. The nurses noticed that the toes of his broken leg were blue in color and insensitive to touch. Yet no action was taken by the hospital in response to this significant observation. Later, nurses reported a foul odor emanating from Darling's room. Again no action was taken other than closing the door to Darling's room to prevent the odor from disturbing other patients. Soon after that, Darling was transferred to Barnes Hospital in St. Louis, where his then-gangrenous leg was amputated.

A malpractice suit was filed by Darling and his family against Dr. Alexander and Charleston Community Memorial Hospital. Dr. Alexander settled out of court, and the case proceeded against the hospital. The hospital argued that the physician, not the hospital, was responsible for the practice and the quality of medicine. Thus the hospital's attorney argued that it was the physician who should be held liable for the bad outcome, not the hospital.

The court rejected that argument and ruled against the hospital. In *Darling v. Charleston Community Memorial Hospital* (1965), it stated the following:

> Present day hospitals, as their manner of operation plainly demonstrates, do far more than furnish facilities for treatment. . . . Certainly the person who avails himself of hospital facilities expects that the hospital will attempt to cure him, not that its nurses or other employees will act on their own responsibility. . . . Licensing, per se, furnished no continuing control with respect to a physician's competence, and, therefore, does not assure the public of quality patient care. *The protection of the public must come from some other authority, and that, in this case, is the hospital board of trustees* [emphasis added].

As can be seen from this ruling, the court held that the *hospital board* had a significant responsibility for the quality of patient care and for the oversight and control of the medical staff and employees. The notion that "T[he] protection of the public must come from . . . the hospital board of trustees" was a significant, if not revolutionary, development in the history of the responsibility for quality.

The *Darling* decision was appealed by the hospital up to the Illinois Supreme Court, which refused to hear the case, letting the judgment of the lower court stand. This ruling had a profound impact on hospitals throughout the country by significantly expanding their responsibility for the quality of care and their liability for failing to reasonably attempt to provide high-quality care.

As stated by Koskoff and Nadeau (1974), the *Darling* case specifically expanded the hospital's responsibility and liability to include the following:

1. The hospital must not allow an independent staff physician to violate a specific hospital requirement for patient safety.
2. The hospital must ensure that its employees will detect apparent dangers to the patient and bring such dangers to the attention of the hospital medical or surgical staff and the administration so that the administration can act to alleviate the danger.
3. The hospital has a duty to supervise the actions of independent staff physicians.

The *Darling* decision also had a profound impact on hospital boards and their responsibility for quality and for meaningful oversight and control of the medical staff. Much of the significance of the *Darling* decision was that it sparked considerable environmental change that significantly expanded the board's responsibility for quality patient care. *Darling* directly caused major changes in state hospital licensing statutes and Joint Commission quality assurance standards, which further heightened the board's responsibility. For example, the first quality assurance standard was published by the Joint Commission in 1966, one year after the *Darling* decision was upheld by the Illinois Supreme Court (Joint Commission on Accreditation of Healthcare Organizations, 1988, p. 12).

A helpful way to understand the significance of the *Darling* decision and the far-reaching changes it caused is to examine these changes graphically. Figure 2-1 shows the legal and conceptual relationship among the hospital governing body (the board), administration, and medical staff as it existed prior to 1965 and the *Darling* decision. The pre-*Darling* responsibility of the hospital board was limited solely to the facility itself, nonmedical services, the equipment, finances, and supplies. The board delegated this responsibility to, and was responsible for overseeing, the hospital administration.

Figure 2-1 is also significant in that it portrays the pre-*Darling* relationship between the board and the medical staff. It shows that prior to 1965 the board did not have organizational authority over the medical staff. In fact, the board and medical staff are seen as coequal organizational bodies with authority over very different areas. Figure 2-1 shows the pre-*Darling* hospital to be a house divided with, at most, a tangential relationship between the board and the medical staff.

Notice that figure 2-1 clearly demonstrates that in the pre-*Darling* hospital the responsibility for the provision and the quality of care lay solely with the medical staff. The board did not have the responsibility

Figure 2-1. Legal Relationships among the Governing Body, Administration, and Medical Staff (pre-1965)

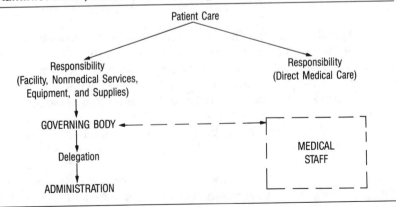

Source: Caniff (1980).

for quality to delegate to the medical staff, nor did the board oversee the medical staff to ensure that they provided quality care. This was very consistent with the law of the time as expressed by the *Pepke v. Grace* and *Schloendorff* decisions, as well as the Minimum Standard of the American College of Surgeons, and the initial *Standards* of the Joint Commission.

The impact of the *Darling* decision can be seen in figure 2-2. The results of the *Darling* decision and the changes in state laws and regulatory requirements that it stimulated strikingly changed the organizational, legal, and conceptual relationship among the hospital governing board, administration, and medical staff. The ultimate responsibility for quality patient care, and indeed everything within the hospital, is plainly seen as resting on the board's shoulders.

In the post-*Darling* hospital depicted in figure 2-2, the board is seen as dividing and delegating responsibility for quality to the hospital administration and the medical staff, but the board retains the ultimate authority and responsibility. Also, the board is now shown as the ultimate authority of the entire hospital, an authority that specifically includes organizational authority over the medical staff. Comparing figure 2-1 to figure 2-2 demonstrates the significant expansion in the hospital board's responsibility for quality of care as well as for the effective (non-"rubber-stamp") oversight of the hospital's medical staff. Even though figure 2-2 shows the legal and conceptual organizational structure of every American hospital today, it does not reflect the actual practice of many, if not most, boards relative to quality and medical staff oversight.

This is not surprising when you consider that the *Darling* decision is a relatively recent one. Thus the implications of implementing the

Figure 2-2. Legal Relationships among the Governing Body, Administration, and Medical Staff (current)

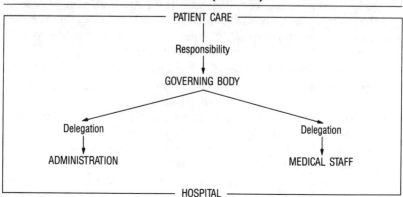

Source: Caniff (1980).

organizational changes mandated by it, along with the many changes it initiated, involve reversing over 200 years of the history of American hospitals and over 4,000 years of historical precedent in the minds of physicians, the public, and hospital trustees.

Conclusion

As this chapter has shown, the concern for quality in health care is by no means a recent development. Yet issues related to quality are so elementary that they indicate that the field of quality is still in its infancy. These issues include how quality is defined, how it is measured, how it can be improved, and who is responsible for it.

The history of the development of the concern for high-quality care has focused on these questions. In fact, the answers to some of these questions have actually changed over time, and it is reasonable to assume that they will continue to change as these important issues receive increasingly closer scrutiny.

Nevertheless, it is imperative that you and your board address these questions now so that your hospital can deliver and demonstrate quality patient care. The remainder of this book will attempt to help you do just that.

□ References

American College of Surgeons. The Minimum Standard of the American College of Surgeons' Hospital Standardization Program. *Bulletin of the American College of Surgeons* 8(4), 1924.

Bing v. Thunig, 2 NY2d 656, 143 NW2d3 163 N.Y.S. 2d3 (1957).

Caniff, Jr., C. E. Responsibilities and relationships of the medical staff, administration, and governing body. Presented at the American Medical Association seminar "Medical Staff: Physician, Friend, or Foe," Chicago, Apr. 24, 1980.

Codman, E. A. *A Study in Hospital Efficiency: The First Five Years.* Boston: Thomas Todd Co., 1916.

Cohen, B. I. Florence Nightingale. *Scientific American* 250(3), Mar. 1984.

Darling v. Charleston Community Memorial Hospital, 33 Ill.2d 326, 211 NE, 2d 253 (1965), *cert. denied* 383 U.S. 946 (1966).

Joint Commission on Accreditation of Healthcare Organizations. *The Joint Commission Guide to Quality Assurance.* Chicago: JCAHO, 1988.

Koskoff, T. I., and Nadeau, T. L. Hospital liability: the emerging standard of care. *Connecticut Bar Journal* 48(305), Sept. 1974.

Kramer, C. *Medical Malpractice.* New York City: Practicing Law Institute, 1976.

Pepke v. Grace, 130 Mich. 493 (1902).

Schloendorff v. Society of New York Hospital, 211 NY125, 105 NE92 (1914).

Chapter 3

Why Hospital Boards Are Responsible for Quality

Introduction

You may have read or heard that boards are ultimately responsible for the quality of care that their hospitals provide. In addition, hospital boards are responsible for the effective functioning of their hospitals' quality assurance programs, medical staff credentialing, and all functions and activities related to quality improvement. Like many trustees, you may have questioned this responsibility and wondered exactly *why* the board is responsible for quality.

This is an important question for you to ask, and an equally important one to have answered to your satisfaction. Before you and your board can truly begin to effectively discharge the responsibility for quality, you and all members of the board must understand and accept why the board has the ultimate responsibility for quality.

As the last chapter indicated, there is a long history of physician accountability and responsibility for quality but a comparatively short history for responsibility of the board. For this and other reasons, many trustees do not fully understand why their board is responsible for quality, let alone how to go about doing something about this responsibility. As you might imagine, the first step for you and your board to achieve effective oversight of the quality that your hospital provides is to reach a shared understanding of exactly why the board has this critically important responsibility.

This chapter will review the reasons you and your board are responsible for the quality of care in your hospital, the medical staff credentialing function, the quality assurance program, and ongoing quality improvement activities. There are four broad, and often overlapping, reasons the board has this responsibility:

1. Moral and ethical obligation
2. Legal accountability
3. Legislative and regulatory requirements that mandate board responsibility and accountability
4. Fiduciary responsibility

Moral and Ethical Obligation

Imagine that you have a legal contract that states that as long as you are a hospital trustee, you and every member of your family must receive all medical and hospital care from your hospital. Neither you nor any of your family could go to another hospital, not even for specialized treatment or surgery for which another hospital was renowned. If that were true, would that in any way increase your interest in ensuring that your hospital consistently delivers high-quality care?

If your answer to that hypothetical question was yes (and whose wouldn't be?), then you can easily begin to understand the ethical and moral obligation of the board to be responsible for quality of care. This is because in a real sense as a trustee you do have such a "social contract" with the community your hospital serves.

The majority of hospital boards are made up of trustees who come from the community served by the hospital, and most boards represent the interests of the community to the hospital and the interests of the hospital to the community. As a result, it is likely that your family, your friends, your neighbors, your business associates, your customers or acquaintances are (or will be) patients served by your hospital. This, combined with the fact that the board is the ultimate authority of the hospital, frames the board's moral and ethical obligation to ensure that quality care is provided to all patients served by the hospital. You would want quality care for yourself or your family; you should also want it for all the hospital's patients.

The board's moral and ethical quality imperative is probably the most important but least considered mandate for the board's duty and responsibility to oversee and ensure the hospital's quality of care. This important obligation can be seen in the board's duty to ensure that the hospital achieves, or constantly strives to achieve, its mission.

Think about your hospital's mission statement or, if it does not quickly come to mind, look it up. If your hospital mission statement is like the vast majority of hospital mission statements in the United States, it stresses that a primary purpose of the hospital is to provide quality care to the patients and the community. The mission statement defines the purpose and direction of the hospital, and the board is charged with ensuring that the hospital strives to achieve and remain true to its mission.

Thus, the mission of the hospital is an ethical and moral mandate for the board. That your hospital's mission statement stresses quality care reflects the board's greater ethical and moral obligation to ensure that the hospital provides quality care to its patients.

It was this ethical and moral obligation that the Illinois court referred to in its ruling in the *Darling* case when it stated that "The protection of the public must come from . . . the hospital board of trustees." In fact, the court took the ethical and moral obligation of the board to be responsible for quality as the basis for establishing a legal duty for board responsibility for quality.

Although the other reasons that follow in this chapter for why the board is responsible for quality may seem more concrete, none is more compelling or more basic than the ethical or moral responsibility of the trustee and the board to make certain that the hospital provides high-quality care. Please think about this crucial reason why you and your board have such a significant responsibility, and then consider it in relation to the question of why you are a trustee of your hospital. Odds are you will recognize that the purpose of trusteeship, the very reason that you are a hospital trustee, is part and parcel of the board's ethical and moral responsibility to ensure that its hospital provides high-quality patient care.

Legal Accountability

As mentioned in chapter 2, the Code of Hammurabi demonstrates the linkage between the responsibility for quality and society's requirement that someone or some group be held accountable for malpractice or substandard care. Chapter 2 also showed how legal decisions in medical malpractice cases helped to frame and define the hospital board's responsibility for the quality of care as well as oversight of the medical staff.

The second reason that the hospital board is responsible for the quality of care comes from the legal accountability of the board as defined in malpractice cases such as *Darling*. Although *Darling* was a landmark decision that framed the board's responsibility for quality care and medical staff oversight, many other rulings in malpractice cases in dozens of states that have reinforced and advanced the board's ultimate authority, accountability, and responsibility for quality. For example, in 1975 the Supreme Court of New Jersey issued a ruling with significant impact on hospital boards in that state. In *Corleto v. Shore Memorial Hospital* the Court ruled that the board of trustees as well as the medical staff could be held legally liable if it could be reasonably shown that any one of them knew that a physician was not competent to practice and was at all responsible for granting privileges to the incompetent physician.

In 1981, the Wisconsin Court of Appeals resoundingly emphasized the hospital board's responsibility for the quality of care and the purposeful oversight of the medical staff in the malpractice case of *Johnson v. Misericordia Community Hospital.* In that case, a physician named Salinsky applied to join the medical staff of Misericordia Community Hospital. In response to a question on his application he stated that his privileges had never been suspended or revoked at another hospital, which was in fact untrue. He also did not answer questions on the application form about the status of his malpractice insurance, leaving them blank. Yet, despite the omission and the false statement in the application, the medical staff recommended and the board approved (or "rubber stamped") Dr. Salinsky's admission to Misericordia's medical staff.

Soon after he was admitted, Dr. Salinsky was elected chief of the medical staff. As a member of the medical staff, he requested privileges in orthopedic surgery. As chief of staff, he *signed off on his own request and recommended to the board that his own request be approved.* The board, clearly operating in the pre-*Darling* "rubber-stamp" mode, approved Dr. Salinsky's request for privileges. Shortly thereafter, while performing orthopedic surgery, Dr. Salinsky severely injured a boy by severing the femoral artery and nerve in his right leg.

A malpractice case was filed against the physician and the hospital and worked its way up to the Wisconsin Court of Appeals, which ruled against Misericordia and Dr. Salinsky. The *Johnson v. Misericordia* case (1980) stated:

> [It is] clear that the medical staff is responsible to the governing body of the hospital for the quality of all medical care provided patients. . . . The [medical] staff must be organized with a proper structure to carry out the role delegated to it by the governing body. *All powers of the medical staff flow from the board of trustees, and the staff must be held accountable for its control of quality. . . . The protection of the public must come from . . . the Hospital Board of Trustees* [emphasis added].

The *Misericordia* ruling relied on the language of the *Darling* decision and went beyond it to demonstrate the board's legal accountability for both the quality of patient care as well as the effective oversight of the medical staff via the medical staff credentialing function.

Many other legal rulings and judgments stemming from malpractice cases have expanded the responsibility of the board for quality care and medical staff oversight. The results of these cases have broadened the duties, responsibilities, and accountability of the hospital and its board that were first hinted at in the *Bing v. Thunig* decision and later framed in the *Darling* decision. One significant effect of these malpractice cases was to establish, expand, and reinforce the ultimate legal responsibility of the hospital board for the quality of care provided by the hospital and for medical staff appointments and privilege delineations.

These cases demonstrate that the board's responsibility includes acting to correct situations where poor quality exists or where physicians are incompetent. Thus the board is not just legally responsible for overseeing the quality of care provided, it must *take* or *direct* action to improve quality or to correct quality-related problems when circumstances warrant.

Literally hundreds of such malpractice cases address the hospital board's responsibility for quality and medical staff oversight spanning the majority of states, and even several protectorates and territories. For purposes of brevity not all cases from all states are listed. However, you may wish to ask your hospital attorney or risk manager to provide you with examples of malpractice cases that are specific to your state to learn legal accountability of the board for quality and medical staff oversight.

Legislative and Regulatory Requirements

In addition to board accountability and responsibility for quality that comes from case law, many requirements from legislative and regulatory bodies require board authority and responsibility for quality and for medical staff oversight. Bodies and agencies issuing such requirements include the Joint Commission on Accreditation of Healthcare Organizations, the federal government, and state legislatures.

The Joint Commission on Accreditation of Healthcare Organizations

The board's responsibility for quality and medical staff credentialing is specifically emphasized by the standards of the Joint Commission on Accreditation of Healthcare Organizations (formerly known as the Joint Commission on Accreditation of Hospitals). Compliance with the standards is necessary for a hospital to receive and maintain accreditation from the Joint Commission.

Emphasis on board responsibility for quality is evident throughout the section of the Joint Commission's 1990 *Accreditation Manual for Hospitals* that addresses the standards and required characteristics for the Governing Body:

> GB.1 An organized governing body, or designated persons so functioning, is responsible for establishing policy, *maintaining quality patient care,* and providing for institutional management and planning [emphasis added].

GB.1.11 The medical staff executive committee makes recommendations *directly to the governing body for its approval* [emphasis
added]. . . . Such recommendations pertain to at least the
following: . . .

GB.1.11.1.2 The mechanism used to review credentials and to delineate individual clinical privileges;

GB.1.11.1.3 Individual medical staff membership;

GB.1.11.1.4 Specific clinical privileges for each eligible individual;

GB.1.11.1.5 The organization of the quality assurance activities of the
medical staff as well as the mechanism used to conduct, evaluate,
and revise such activities; . . .

The Governing Body section of the Joint Commission's accreditation
manual outlines additional standards and required characteristics that
further stress overall and specific board responsibilities for quality:

GB.1.15 The governing body requires a process . . . designed to
assure that all individuals who provide patient care services, but who
are not subject to the medical staff privilege delineation process, are
competent to provide such services . . .

GB.1.16 The governing body requires mechanisms to assure the provision of one level of patient care in the hospital . . .

GB.1.18 The governing body provides for resources and support systems for the quality assurance functions and risk management functions related to patient care and safety . . .

GB.3.2 All members of the governing body are provided information relating to the governing body's responsibility for quality care
and the hospital's quality assurance program.

These standards and required characteristics promulgated by the Joint
Commission are quite pointed in framing several responsibilities, duties,
and functions of the board that relate to the issues of quality of care,
quality assurance, and medical staff credentialing.

It is worth noting, however, that these specific Governing Body standards and required characteristics were implemented only relatively
recently. The "Governing Body" chapter of standards became effective
for accreditation purposes on April 1, 1984. More specifically, the requirement that the board provide support to the quality assurance and risk
management functions (GB.1.18) was implemented for accreditation purposes only on January 1, 1989. This further demonstrates the relatively

new emphasis on the board's responsibility and authority for quality that was addressed in chapter 2.

The Joint Commission also publishes "scoring guidelines," which its surveyors use as practical guidelines to assess a hospital's level of compliance with the standards and the required characteristics of the standards. The Joint Commission required characteristic GB.1.18 is significant not only for its recency, but also in terms of what it specifically requires regarding board support for quality assurance and risk management. The Joint Commission 1990 scoring guidelines for GB.1.18 state in part:

Elements of Satisfactory Performance

1. The governing body requires performance of and has delegated responsibility for the following quality assurance/risk management functions:
   - Identification of general clinical areas that represent actual or potential sources of patient injury
   - Development and use of an indicator based approach to identifying and evaluating individual cases of undesirable or adverse patient-care occurrences within the general clinical areas
   - Resolution of clinical problems disclosed through data evaluation
   - Provision of education for all staff on approaches to reducing or eliminating potential clinical sources of patient injury
2. The governing body receives reports at least every six months on:
   - The frequency, severity, and causes of undesirable or adverse patient-care occurrences; and
   - Actions taken and the results of actions taken to reduce the occurrences' frequency and severity or to eliminate their causes.

The Joint Commission is the primary American voluntary accreditation agency for hospitals. The emphasis placed by the Joint Commission on the responsibility of the hospital board for the hospital's quality, quality assurance program and related activities, and medical staff credentialing activities is therefore significant.

The Federal Government

The federal government, through its Medicare program, is responsible for a substantial portion of most hospitals' revenues. To receive Medicare reimbursement, a hospital must comply with the requirements set forth by the government in a document that is essentially a contract, called Conditions of Participation in the Medicare Program (Anthony and Singer, 1989, p. 19). The Conditions of Participation, like the Joint Commission, also requires board responsibility for quality, and thus represents another legislative and regulatory mandate for board oversight of quality.

Anthony and Singer also point out that to be eligible for Medicare reimbursement, a hospital must have an effective governing body that is the ultimate legal authority of the hospital; and further, that the board must ensure that the medical staff is accountable directly to the board for the quality of care.

State Licensure Laws and Statutes

In addition to the requirements of the Joint Commission and the Conditions of Participation in the Medicare Program, other legislative and regulatory requirements mandate board responsibility for quality. Hospital licensure laws in all 50 states address in one form or another the responsibility of the hospital board for quality and for oversight of the medical staff.

For example, note the following language from the hospital licensing statute enacted by the Michigan legislature in 1968, three years after the *Darling* decision (Kitch, 1986):

> The governing body of each hospital shall be responsible for . . . , the selection of the medical staff, and the quality of care rendered in the hospital. The governing body shall . . . , insure that physicians admitted to practice in the hospital are granted hospital privileges consistent with their individual training, experience and other qualifications; and insure that physicians admitted to practice in the hospital are organized into a medical staff in such a manner as to effectively review the professional practices of the hospital for the purposes of reducing morbidity and mortality. . . .

It is interesting to note that this language comes from the same state where the *Pepke v. Grace* decision was handed down by the Michigan Supreme Court in 1902. That comparison aside, this and other state hospital licensure laws and statutes are quite significant in that they specify ultimate responsibility and authority of the board for quality of care and effective oversight of the medical staff.

Again, space does not permit a listing of the relevant portions of all 50 state hospital licensure laws and statutes here. It is a worthwhile exercise, however, to read the law from your own state to get a very real sense of your hospital board's specific legal duty and authority for quality. Toward that end, you might ask your hospital chief executive officer or hospital attorney to obtain a copy of the hospital licensure law (or equivalent) specific to your state and to highlight the portion relating to the board's responsibilities for you and the entire board to read.

Fiduciary Responsibility

Preceding sections of this chapter may have convinced you of the reality and significance of board responsibility for quality and medical staff oversight. You may have found the ethical and moral obligation, the legal accountability, and the legislative and regulatory requirements all to be persuasive arguments. Unfortunately, many trustees, not persuaded by these arguments, do not regard quality to be the responsibility of the board in any real or meaningful way and often dismiss them even after detailed review. The primary responsibility of the board—the one that transcends all others, these trustees will argue—is the board's fiduciary responsibility; that is, the board's responsibility to exercise diligent and effective financial oversight of the hospital. Although the board's financial responsibility is obviously a critically important one, the argument that it is the *only* real responsibility or even the *single most important* responsibility of the board engenders a complacent and dangerous attitude toward the board's responsibility for quality.

Often, trustees who hold that perspective will express it in the following way: "The board takes care of finance, and the medical staff takes care of quality." This is in fact the way it actually *used to be* (as evidenced by figure 2-1 in chapter 2). This division of responsibility was also in many instances the cause of substandard care and patient injury. The perspective that quality is the medical staff's job and finance is the board's job is really an abdication of the board's responsibility and a conceptual throwback to the pre-*Darling* days of hospital organization.

This is such a common misconception among trustees, however, that to emphasize the board's responsibility for quality, the responsibility is often compared in importance to the board's financial responsibility. For example, the American Hospital Association in its 1987 *Guidelines: Physician Involvement in Governance of Health Care Institutions* states:

> A primary responsibility of a hospital governing board is to achieve and maintain high-quality patient care. Boards have as much responsibility for the quality of health services delivered as they have for an institution's financial affairs.

Yet simply restating the concept that quality is an important board responsibility will not convince those trustees who feel "finance is the board's responsibility, quality is the medical staff's." Instead, it is necessary to demonstrate that one key reason boards must be concerned with quality is *precisely because* they have financial responsibility for their hospital.

There is a definite relationship between a hospital's quality of care and its financial viability. In fact, a hospital that provides poor-quality care will suffer for it financially, whereas a hospital that provides high-quality care will realize financial benefits. Thus a trustee or board that focuses on finance as the board's key responsibility *must* become concerned with quality to achieve and maintain financial viability.

Poor-quality care can have significant negative impact on a hospital's finances in at least three ways:

1. It can drive patients away from the hospital and toward competing hospitals.
2. It can increase the hospital's exposure to loss from malpractice liability.
3. It generally costs a hospital more money to provide poor-quality care and thus can reduce operating margins.

Preventing Loss of Market Share

Ask yourself these questions: Would you go to a hospital if you knew that it did not provide high-quality care? Given the choice between two hospitals, would you choose the one that provided substandard care? Most likely you would answer no to both questions, just as the majority of the public probably would. The issue is whether public perceptions of the quality of care a hospital provides will influence people's choice of a hospital.

An article in the *Journal of the American Medical Association* presented the findings of research into that very question. The question posed by the researchers was: Does quality influence the choice of hospital? They examined data from California in 1983, which is a interesting time because that was *before* significant quality data on hospitals were released to the public. Even so, the researchers concluded, "The results suggest that quality played an important role in choices among hospitals even before explicit data were widely available" (Luft, 1990).

The environment today is much different than in 1983. Today's public is constantly presented with explicit data that purport to demonstrate the quality, or lack thereof, of particular hospitals. In fact, the data often are used to compare quality among hospitals. Such data come from the federal government mortality rates for Medicare patients, from peer review organizations, from the media, and even from hospital regulators. Table 3-1 presents just such a comparison of hospital mortality rates for cardiac surgery that appeared in an article in the *Wall Street Journal* (Schiffman, 1990).

Clearly the information presented in table 3-1 might have an impact on a patient's choice of hospital for cardiac bypass surgery. Thus the hospitals with the lowest mortality rates (or, as the chart and the article imply, the best "quality") might see an increase in business for this and other procedures, whereas the hospitals with the highest mortality (or worst "quality") might see a significant decrease in business—not just for that one procedure, but overall. So, quality can affect a hospital's financial position by either attracting or repelling patients and thus can increase or decrease revenues flowing to the hospital.

Minimizing Exposure to Loss from Malpractice Liability

Another way that quality can affect a hospital's finances is by way of malpractice costs. (Remember, the link between quality and malpractice goes back 4,000 years to Hammurabi.) If a hospital is not providing quality care, or, rather, is providing poor-quality care, that hospital likely will be at increased risk of being sued for malpractice. This in turn will cost the hospital money in several ways.

Table 3-1.   Hospitals with the Highest and Lowest 1987 Mortality Rates for Coronary-Artery Bypass Surgery on Medicare Patients

Hospital	Mortality Rate	Annual Number of Procedures
Lowest Mortality Rate		
Henry Ford (Detroit)	0.00%	89
Terrebonne (Houma, LA)	0.00	78
Grossmont District (La Mesa, CA)	0.00	68
Montana Deaconess (Great Falls, MT)	0.00	66
University of California (San Diego)	0.00	44
Missouri Baptist (St. Louis)	0.46	218
Mother Frances (Tyler, TX)	0.79	127
West Houston (Houston)	0.91	110
Henricos Doctors (Richmond, VA)	1.03	195
St. Marys (Huntington, WV)	1.05	95
Theda Clark (Neenah, WI)	1.20	83
Southern Baptist (New Orleans)	1.64	61
Highest Mortality Rate		
University of Chicago (Chicago)	22.81%	57
Mt. Carmel Health (Columbus, OH)	22.37	152
Parkland (Dallas)	21.88	32
St. Joseph (Burbank, CA)	20.00	70
Cleveland Metro (Cleveland)	20.00	45
Jackson (Miami)	19.51	41
St. Francis (Miami Beach, FL)	19.40	67
White (Los Angeles)	19.35	31
Houston Northwest (Houston)	18.18	33
St. Paul Ramsey (St. Paul, MN)	17.95	39
Memorial (Corpus Christi, TX)	17.95	39

Source: Schiffman (1990). Reprinted by permission of the *Wall Street Journal*, ©1990 Dow Jones & Company, Inc. All Rights Reserved Worldwide.

Note: Includes only hospitals performing at least 30 procedures a year.

If the hospital is sued for malpractice and loses, it may have to pay part of the judgment. Additionally, its malpractice insurance costs will rise in response. Even if the hospital is sued and wins, its insurance costs will likely rise. As was demonstrated in chapter 2, malpractice cases o. • .n involve failure of a hospital and its board to effectively oversee the hospital's quality and performance of its medical staff. Thus a fairly typical result of poor quality – malpractice claims and lawsuits – can affect a hospital's finances and hurt its bottom line.

Trimming Operating Expenses

Another reason that trustees concerned solely with hospital finances should be concerned also with hospital quality is that substandard care is more expensive to provide than is high-quality care. This concept has been demonstrated in other industries for years and has recently surfaced in the hospital field.

To demonstrate this, consider a study conducted in 1989 that reviewed 1 million patients treated in 1987 in New Jersey's acute care hospitals. As a measure of quality, the researchers compared each hospital's mortality rate for five categories of medical and surgical patients to a predetermined standard. They demonstrated that the hospitals that had the lowest mortality rates and highest quality in spinal, head, and neck surgery spent an average of 34 percent less on the care of those patients than did the hospitals with the highest mortality rates and lowest quality. The same pattern was evident for other procedures as well. The study also demonstrated that the hospitals providing the highest-quality care in these areas also had a much greater share of the market than did those hospitals with poorer-quality care (Binns and Early, 1989; Schiffman, 1989).

The researchers (Binns and Early, 1989) in fact addressed the very issue of the relationship between quality and finance and spoke to the need of the board to be concerned with quality as a critical determinant of the hospital's financial viability:

> The principal finding from all of the LHS [Lexecon Health Service] research is that high quality outcomes are associated with lower-cost care. Not only are high quality outcomes a potential marketing tool for hospitals, but the savings from avoiding complications and death will drop to a hospital's bottom line. . . .

To emphasize the financial impact of poor quality consider the example of nosocomial infections. A *nosocomial infection* is generally defined as an infection acquired in the hospital. Nosocomial infections and their control are discussed in greater depth later in this book. Here, nosocomial infections are discussed simply in the context of the costs of poor quality.

Holzman (1988) demonstrates that the average nonfatal nosocomial infection costs about $1,800 to treat. Note that in the majority of cases the *hospital*, not the patient or third-party payer, absorbs the cost of the nosocomial infection. Armed with this information, it is now possible to perform a simple equation to demonstrate the significant financial impact of poor-quality care.

Find out what your hospital's annual nosocomial infection rate is and what the annual discharges of the hospital are. Then perform this equation:

Nosocomial infection rate × Annual hospital discharges
× $1,800
= Dollar cost to hospital resulting from nosocomial infections

Now perform the equation again with the nosocomial infection rate *reduced* by 1 percent. Note the amount of money that your hospital would save annually if it could reduce its nosocomial infection rate by 1 percent. Nosocomial infections are one small component of a hospital's overall quality of care. Yet the financial impact of these infections on your hospital's bottom line is easy to see. The same logic, and negative financial impact, for other examples of poor quality of care also applies.

As you can see, malpractice losses, lost market share, and higher operating costs can be consequences of poor-quality care; thus quality of care has a very definite financial impact on the hospital. Consequently, a trustee who regards the primary responsibility of the hospital board to be financial therefore *must* become concerned about quality.

Conclusion

You and all members of your board share a very important responsibility for the quality of care provided by the hospital your board governs. This may at first seem to you and the other trustees of your board an awesome and incomprehensible obligation. Nevertheless, it is a very real and important responsibility of your board, one that becomes more understandable as you consider the reasons *why* the board has this responsibility.

Once you understand this, the next step is to make certain that the management and medical staff also understand why the board is responsible for quality and what imperatives drive and define that responsibility. Only after this shared understanding is achieved can you and your board begin to address *how* to effectively discharge the board's responsibility for quality of patient care.

☐ References

American Hospital Association. *Guidelines: Physician Involvement in Governance of Health Care Institutions.* Chicago: AHA, 1987.

Anthony, M. F., and Singer, L. E. The legal basis of the board's quality assurance duties. *Trustee,* 42(1):2, 19, Jan. 1989.

Binns, G. S., and Early, J. F. Hospital care: frontiers in managing quality. *Juran Report,* No. 10, Autumn 1989.

Corleto v. Shore Memorial Hospital, 350 A2d 534 (NJ 1975).

Holzman, D. The sickly side of hospital stays. *Insight,* Apr. 18, 1988.

Johnson v. Misericordia Community Hospital, 294 NW 2d 501 (1980), Wisc. Court of Appeals.

Joint Commission on Accreditation of Healthcare Organizations. *Accreditation Manual for Hospitals.* Chicago: JCAHO, 1990.

Joint Commission on Accreditation of Healthcare Organizations. *Scoring Guidelines for Hospital Risk Management Activities.* Chicago: JCAHO, 1990.

Kitch, R. A. *Legal Liability in Conjunction with Credentialing* (pamphlet). Detroit: Kitch, Saurbier, Drutchas, Wagner & Kenney, P.C., Nov. 1986.

Luft, H. S., Garnick, D. W., Mark, D. H., and others. Does quality influence choice of hospital? *Journal of the American Medical Association* 263(21):2899–2906, June 6, 1990.

Schiffman, J. R. Practice Makes Better [special section on medicine and health]. *Wall Street Journal,* May 11, 1990.

Schiffman, J. R. Health costs: high costs, quality don't go hand in hand. *Wall Street Journal,* Nov. 10, 1989, p. B1.

Chapter 4

Becoming Comfortable with the Basics of Quality

Introduction

Chapter 3 may have helped convince you *why* your board has significant responsibility for the quality of care your hospital provides. Odds are, however, that even if you are convinced about this responsibility, you and the other members of your board may not be completely comfortable with it.

One reason for your discomfort probably rests with the vagueness of the issue of quality. What is quality? How is it measured? What is quality assurance? These may be some of the questions that need to be addressed so that you and your board can begin to feel comfortable with the issue of quality. For some of these questions there are no firm answers; for others, the answers are ever evolving.

It is not critically important that these questions have solid answers for you and your board to effectively oversee quality in your hospital. What is important is that you and your board ask the questions and then discuss them. This discussion should expand to include your hospital management and medical staff leadership.

Asking and discussing the questions will generate answers that have specific meaning for you, your medical staff, and your hospital. This chapter will address these questions, pose issues for your consideration, and, where they exist, provide answers to make you and the other members of your board more comfortable with quality and its many attendant issues.

What Is Quality?

Before you and your board can do anything to improve the quality of care your hospital delivers or to maintain a high level of quality care, you must have a sense of what you are talking about. What *is* quality, anyway?

There is no question that quality is an elusive concept to grasp. One reason for this is that it is so hard to define, usually because it often means very different things to different people. Yet developing a definition of quality is not so difficult; the trick is coming up with a definition that is *measurable*.

Remember Hammurabi's "definition" of quality? Essentially, health care quality for him involved not causing injuries, specifically a physician not causing death or the loss of an eye in a free man. You probably think that in your hospital there is much more to quality, and of course you are right. There is no question that Hammurabi's definition of quality is limited and limiting. The one advantage it has, however, is that his definition is easily measured.

The challenge, then, is to develop a working definition of quality that facilitates its measurement. Quality must be measurable to allow your board and hospital to determine whether good, poor, or fair quality is being delivered, as well to ascertain whether quality is being improved.

Perhaps the best way to conceptualize as well as define quality is to consider it in terms of the many *perspectives* of quality. For example, there is the medical perspective. This is the professional perspective of the physicians on your medical staff and probably relates to issues such as the degree to which care meets accepted standards or patterns of practice as defined by clinical research and medical professional societies.

There is also the patient or consumer perspective. Patients may define quality less in terms of clinical standards or outcomes and more in terms of attentiveness of the nurses and hospital staff, clarity of communication, waiting times, and amenities such as hospital environment and food.

The perspective of the patients of your hospital will probably be very different from the perspective of the medical staff regarding what quality is. Does this mean that only one of these two perspectives can actually relate to quality, that there is only one valid perspective?

Consider the following hypothetical situation that is frequently presented to trustees. You are in a board meeting when, by chance, the board is presented with two quality-related reports. The first is from the chief of the medical staff, who reports on the results of a detailed and elegant six-month study of the quality of medical care in your hospital's emergency department. The study showed that, from a medical/clinical perspective, the quality of care in the emergency room (ER) was very high, excellent in fact. Further, the study was examined by an outside researcher who stated that its results were valid, reliable, and meaningful.

The second report is from the patient representative, who reports that the hospital has known for years that the emergency room generates by far the largest number of patient complaints compared to any other area. On the basis of this knowledge, a six-month study of patient perceptions of quality in the ER was conducted. The results of the study clearly showed that the patients regard the quality of care in the ER as being terrible. This study has also been externally reviewed, and its results are also valid, reliable, and meaningful.

Now the results of the two studies are left for your board to consider relative to each other. The physicians say the medical/clinical care is excellent in the ER, whereas the patients say that the quality of ER care is terrible. It is now time for you and the board to answer a simple question: Just what exactly *is* the level of quality of care in the ER?

How did you answer the hypothetical question? Did you (as many trustees have) say that the care is excellent? Did you (as many other trustees have) say that the care is terrible? Did you come up with yet another answer?

Yes, another answer is possible; in fact it is the right answer and one given by a fair number of trustees. That answer is that the quality of care in the ER is *both* excellent and terrible. It is excellent from the medical/clinical perspective but terrible from the patient perspective. In other words, the overall quality of care in the ER has components of excellence and components of inadequacy.

This is more than a trick question because it strikes at the very heart of defining quality. Had your board in this hypothetical situation defined quality solely from the medical/clinical perspective, you would have answered that the quality of care in the ER was excellent. More important, you most probably would have disregarded the patients' perceptions of the ER quality and would not have take action to address them.

Conversely, had your board taken only the patients' perspective as defining quality, you would have viewed the quality of care in the ER as being terrible. As a result, your board might have mandated action to improve those characteristics in the ER that upset the patients. Although this may be appropriate action, your board would probably have disregarded the physicians' perspective and would not have given them positive reinforcement for delivering high-quality clinical care.

Thus the perspectives of quality that you and your board regard as being important will actually frame your practical definition of quality. In the hypothetical situation just described, a board that included both the medical/clinical perspective *and* the patient perspective in its overall view of quality would have accepted and responded to both studies. The answer that the ER has both components of excellent and terrible quality allows the board and the hospital to do several important things relating to achieving and maintaining high-quality care. It allows them the opportunity to recognize and reward those who contributed to the excellent medical ER quality and to take steps to maintain that excellent care.

It also enables them to respond to the problems that are negatively affecting the perceptions of the patients and to correct them so as to improve the patients' perceptions.

The concept of combining accepted perspectives of quality to attain a practical definition of quality is, for a board and its hospital, a very important and powerful one. This is because the information that flows to a board about quality will be structured and influenced by its accepted quality perspectives. If a board chooses only one perspective of quality, it will likely receive information only on that single, limited and limiting, perspective of quality.

Equally important, if a board does not make explicit choices about which perspectives of quality it and the hospital value, then its perspectives of quality, and thus its definition of quality, will be determined solely by the information about quality that is sent to the board. Thus if a board is sent only that information relating to the hospital's compliance with the Joint Commission on Accreditation of Healthcare Organizations standards, then the board will define quality simply as meeting Joint Commission standards and maintaining accreditation.

Unfortunately, the situation where the information sent to a board actually structures the board's definition of quality is a very common one. Instead of the tail wagging the dog, so to speak, the board should determine which perspectives of quality it values, develop a specific definition of quality, and then request information that relates to all the quality perspectives it has chosen. This concept simply breaks down to:

1. Identifying which perspectives of quality your board and hospital value
2. Combining all the perspectives into a definition of quality that is specific to your hospital
3. Regularly receiving information that allows the board to determine and address the various levels of quality by each different perspective of quality

In this way quality is not defined as some academic, elusive, or ethereal concept but as a practical and workable statement. In turn, this quality statement will guide the quality assurance and quality improvement activities of the hospital and the board.

So, based on the information it receives and responds to regarding quality, what perspectives of quality does your board value? What perspectives of hospital quality do *you* value? No matter what you answer, it is critical that you and your board realize that no single perspective of quality determines the final and complete definition of quality.

There are many perspectives of quality, and they can be grouped into many categories. One way of grouping them is by internal and external perspectives. *Internal perspectives* of quality relate to those perspectives and information streams that originate from within the hospital. *External perspectives* of quality, obviously, are those that come from outside the hospital. Figure 4-1 presents many different perspectives of quality divided into internal and external categories.

The perspectives of quality presented in figure 4-1 are by no means an exhaustive listing. In fact, you may identify perspectives missing from either the internal or external list. Conversely, you and your board may not view all the perspectives shown as being meaningful or appropriate.

What is important is for you and your board to develop your own list of perspectives of quality, ones that you value. Once the list is developed, the various items should be prioritized to identify those perspectives that are regarded as most important. By doing so you will be constructing a broad definition of quality that is measurable by each specific perspective or component of quality. Further, you will have developed a definition that has specific meaning for your board and hospital.

As a general rule, the more perspectives incorporated into a definition of quality, the more meaningful and measurable that definition will be. Also, an internally developed definition will have more meaning and utility than an externally developed one. In other words, your board

Figure 4-1. Internal and External Perspectives of Quality

Internal Perspectives

Medical/clinical
Patients/consumers
Staff and employees
Medical staff
Management
Visitors, family, vendors
Financial (utilization management)—the cost of care
Others?

External Perspectives

Joint Commission on Accreditation of Healthcare Organizations
The federal government (via Medicare)
Peer review organizations
State hospital licensing agencies
Third-party payers
The community
The media
Hospital insurers
Malpractice attorneys
Statistical and demographic norms
Others?

should develop its own definition of quality rather than importing an external one that may not be meaningful or measurable for your hospital.

Quality is obviously difficult to define in a concise and measurable fashion. Nevertheless, quality must be defined and the definition clearly understood by your board, medical staff, and management if any efforts to measure and improve quality are to succeed. The quality perspective approach to constructing a definition of quality has several advantages and is a good first step. More specific ways of defining quality in relation to the various perspectives of quality will be discussed throughout the rest of this book.

How Quality Is Measured

To track the effectiveness of the hospital's quality assurance and quality improvement activities, the board must know the basics of how quality is measured. This will also help you and members of your board become more comfortable and conversant in the area of quality. These basics will apply to the vast majority of the perspectives of quality, especially the medical/clinical ones.

Structure, Process, and Outcome

There are three basic components of quality measurement: structure, process, and outcome (Donabedian, 1980). All three will be discussed in this section, as well as how they can be used by the board in overseeing hospital quality.

Structure relates to the condition of the physical facility of the hospital—integrity of equipment and quality of supplies. *Process* involves how the care is actually delivered and relates to things such as staffing patterns and training; how policies and procedures are developed and implemented; and the actual technique of the various medical, nursing, and other diagnostic and therapeutic procedures performed. *Outcome*, on the other hand, involves the actual condition of the patient following a hospital-related action (or inaction) such as administering medication, performing a procedure, or making (or failing to make) a diagnosis. It is important for your board to realize that outcome does not apply only to a patient's condition upon discharge from the hospital; a patient can have several different outcomes during hospitalization, another at discharge, and still more outcomes after leaving the hospital.

It is important for you and your board to understand the distinctions between structure, process, and outcome in quality, as well as their interrelationships. This ensures that your hospital's quality assessment and improvement activities are focused appropriately and are instrumental in improving the quality of care.

To clarify the distinction between structure, process, and outcome, consider this common flaw in logic that was applied to hospital quality assurance programs in the late 1970s. It was thought then that there was a linear, cause-and-effect relationship between structure and process, and outcome. That relationship can be expressed in the following equation:

$$Structure + Process = Outcome$$

Basically that meant that if a hospital had good structure and good process it would *necessarily* have good outcome. That would be like saying:

> We have a brand-new hospital with all new state-of-the-art equipment (a structure statement).
> *Plus* we have a medical staff that trained at top-notch medical schools, finished in the top of their classes, and are all board certified; and we have a first-rate nursing staff that follows policies and procedures to the letter (a process statement).
> *Therefore* we must be providing high-quality care (an outcome statement).

Although that may seem like a reasonable statement, the problem with it is that it *assumes* that the outcome of a hospital's care is good.

In fact, there is not a universal linear, cause-and-effect relationship between structure, process, and outcome. That is, it is possible to have good structure and good process, but still have bad outcome. Conversely, it is possible to have bad structure and bad process, and yet have good outcome. The only way to really know is to *measure the outcome*.

Problems in Measuring Outcome

The problem with many hospital quality assurance programs is that they measure structure and process but not outcome. This has occurred over the years (and still occurs in many hospitals) for several reasons. First, it is easier to measure structure and process than it is to measure outcome. This is because outcomes are difficult to define and measure in the aggregate, because all patients are different.

For example, a group of patients may all be diagnosed as having acute myocardial infarction (heart attack), but some will be sicker than others. Now, perhaps some physicians always treat the most seriously ill patients; those physicians will probably show a much higher mortality rate than the physicians who usually treat the patients with mild heart attacks. How, then, can their outcomes be fairly aggregated, analyzed, and compared? This issue can be addressed by adjusting for the *severity of illness*.

Severity of illness adjustment systems that facilitate the analysis of outcomes are a relatively recent development, are somewhat complicated,
and are still being refined.

A second problem that inhibits the measurement of outcome in many
hospitals is that it may be threatening to members of the medical and
hospital staff to have their patients' outcomes assessed, as it may identify problems with the practitioners who provided the care. This fear
on the part of physicians and hospital staff that quality assurance is a
"witch-hunt" or that its sole purpose is to "get" someone is one of the
most common and pervasive barriers to effective quality assurance programs. To overcome this problem, quality assurance programs must
include *rewards and recognition* for high-quality care, as well as corrective action for problematic care. Does your hospital's quality assurance
program reward or recognize individuals or departments that are providing high-quality care?

For these and other reasons, it is important that your board make
certain that the majority of the hospital quality assessment and improvement activities focus on *outcome of care*. The reluctance of the hospital
field in the past to measure and improve outcome is the primary reason
the federal government is focusing attention on outcome by annually
releasing individual hospital Medicare mortality data to the public. It
is also the reason that the Joint Commission and other regulators and
third-party payers are stressing a focus on outcome.

If problems are identified in outcome of care, the way to correct those
problems and improve the care (it is important to stress that so-called
problem-free care can also be improved) may indeed be to make changes
in structure and process. However, instead of focusing on the assessment of structure and process and *assuming* their effect on outcome, it
is far better to assess the actual outcome and then look for the root causes
of poor outcome, or for ways to improve acceptable outcome.

Other Aspects of Measuring Quality

Structure, process, and outcome are the three broad components of quality. Once you and your board are comfortable with those concepts, it
is useful to consider the measurement of quality from another perspective: the time frames of quality measurement. There are three time frames
of quality measurement: retrospective, concurrent, and prospective.

It will help your board's understanding of quality, as well as improve
the effectiveness of your board's oversight of its hospital's quality, to
understand the time frames of quality measurement and improvement,
as well as the relative strengths and weaknesses of each. In fact, one
of the board's most important contributions to high-quality care in its

hospital stems from its understanding of the distinction among and use of the various time frames of quality measurement.

Retrospective Review

As you may recall from chapter 2, Florence Nightingale developed and advanced the use of retrospective review to improve the quality of care. *Retrospective reviews* are simply those activities that measure care that was provided in the past, usually to patients who have been discharged from the hospital. The purpose of retrospective review is to identify elements of that care that can be improved, or problems in the care. That information is then analyzed to implement current action to improve the care or to correct the problems from that point in time forward.

Retrospective review of quality can be a powerful and useful tool in your hospital's quality assurance and improvement program. However, retrospective review has a major limitation, the *feedback loop.* That is, from the time a problem occurs to the time the problem is identified to the time the problem is corrected takes too long. This means that while a component of past care, for example, abdominal surgery, is being investigated retrospectively, patients currently undergoing abdominal surgery may be receiving poor-quality care. The retrospective review will not in any way improve the care of these patients but may improve the care of future patients.

Retrospective reviews are most appropriate when they involve complicated issues having many variables and including large numbers of patients over long periods of time. You should understand that the use of retrospective review will always have a place in your hospital's quality assurance and improvement program, but that it should not be the *only* methodological time frame used. In fact, if retrospective review is the predominant form of quality investigation in your hospital's quality improvement efforts, it should be deemphasized in favor of concurrent review.

Concurrent Review

Concurrent review is generally defined as the assessment of care *as it is being delivered* (Orlikoff, 1990, p.48). Obviously this is not always practical or possible, so an excellent working definition of concurrent review is the assessment of care *while the patient is still in the hospital,* or, assessing the patient's care within 24 hours after it was delivered, for example (Longo and others, 1989, p. 189). The clear advantage of concurrent review is the short feedback loop, that is, the short period from the time patient care is provided to the time that care is assessed and, if problems or opportunities for improvement are found, improved.

To understand the value and power of effective concurrent review in relation to retrospective review, consider this example: You are scheduled to undergo a surgical procedure on a Tuesday. On the preceding Monday, another patient underwent the same procedure conducted in the same surgical suite by the same surgeon and same surgical team who will perform your surgery. Unfortunately for that patient, something went wrong and the patient was injured. Now, under a retrospective system of review, that patient's care will not be assessed until at least 30 days have passed. If the patient's injury was caused by a preventable event or correctable behavior, that will be determined 30 days later, *which is 29 days after your surgical procedure.* In other words, the massive machinery of retrospective review, which probably would eventually correct the problem, would not help improve your care or prevent that same injury from happening to you.

Now consider the same situation but in a hospital where concurrent review is routinely conducted. After the patient's surgery and subsequent injury on Monday, that patient's care would be closely examined soon after the injury. If the injury was caused by a preventable or correctable variable, then corrective action would be implemented right then and there, so that when you are wheeled into the surgical suite on Tuesday, odds of your experiencing that same injury have been minimized or eliminated. Thus as a result of concurrent review conducted yesterday, you would benefit from higher-quality care today.

In many hospitals, major efforts are under way to move the quality review activities away from retrospective review and toward concurrent review. If your hospital is not one of those hospitals, it should be. Your chief executive officer or quality assurance professional can provide your board with examples of the types of concurrent reviews being conducted in your hospital, as well as the relative ratio of use of retrospective review to concurrent review in your hospital. Your board, CEO, and quality assurance professional can determine a goal for this; for example, no more than 60 percent of all the hospital's quality assessment activities will be based on retrospective review. Your board can and should support the movement toward concurrent review of quality in your hospital.

Do remember, however, that complete elimination of retrospective review should *not* be a goal. In fact, retrospective review may still be the workhorse of your hospital's quality assurance and improvement program, as indicated by the sample goal in the previous paragraph. Retrospective review is valuable if it is not overused. The trick is to make certain that your hospital is not overusing it. Some hospitals rely on retrospective review for almost 100 percent of their quality assurance activities, and that is much too high. What percent of quality assurance activities are based on retrospective review in your hospital?

Prospective Review

The concept of prospective review is somewhat confusing. After all, *prospective* means "in the future" and *review* means "in the past." (Remember, even concurrent review is conducted slightly *after* the care is delivered, so it could technically be called retrospective.)

Actually, *prospective review* (and prospective quality assurance and improvement) is defined simply as the review of intended care. In other words, the prospective approach to quality simply means examining new procedures, new techniques, or policies for using new equipment *before* they are operationally implemented. This prospective approach allows a hospital to make certain that all potential problems and avenues for improving care are identified and implemented to *prevent* injuries or quality problems from occurring.

Interestingly, prospective quality assurance tends to occur at the medical and nursing departmental levels but is rarely integrated into the quality assurance and improvement program or even recognized by it. This is most unfortunate because prospective quality assurance is a very powerful approach to improving quality of care and preventing quality-related problems. It is so powerful, in fact, that *your board should actually perform prospective quality assurance.* Unlike retrospective and concurrent quality reviews, which the board does not do but rather makes certain gets done appropriately, the hospital board can and should *do* prospective quality assurance. How can your board actually "do" prospective quality assurance? By integrating quality issues into the majority of decisions your board makes.

For example, your board routinely makes decisions about your hospital and its affairs. These probably include decisions about new business activities (managed care, hospital-sponsored home care, ambulatory surgery centers, and so forth). Your board may also make decisions regarding the purchase of new equipment (laser surgery devices or scanning and imaging devices).

Think about the last time your board made such decisions. If yours is like most boards, it probably considered the financial implications of the decision, such as the capital requirements and the projected return on investment. Your board even may have considered or reviewed marketing plans for the new venture, equipment, or procedure. All that is fine, but did your board consider the new venture or activity in terms of quality?

Very few boards consider how a new venture or activity will be integrated into the hospital's quality assurance and improvement program, or its potential impact on the quality of patient care. This is a natural but very unfortunate extension of the belief of many trustees that "the board takes care of finance, but someone else—like the medical staff—takes care of quality."

Prospective review of the quality implications of such a decision at the board level is quite similar in concept and conduct to the board's review of the financial implications of the decision. The board does not actually *develop* a quality plan for the new venture any more than it develops a financial plan. Instead, the board *reviews* the quality plan, just as it does the financial plan.

By insisting that a quality plan, presented to the board prior to all major decisions, is made a routine part of the board's decision-making process, your board will actually be "doing" prospective quality assurance. The board should get a quality plan for any decision that will in any way affect the way care is provided to patients. A good rule of thumb is that if a decision is important enough to warrant a financial plan for board review, it probably also merits a quality plan.

The quality plan should outline how the new venture, equipment, or procedure will be integrated into the hospital's quality assurance program. It should clearly demonstrate that professionals have given thought to all the possible things that could go wrong with the new activity, and that they have developed preventive strategies and contingency measures for appropriate and quick response.

One big problem with retrospective review is that it has created a mind-set of "we will fix it only if it breaks" or "if it ain't broke, don't fix it." The problem with that thinking is that it forces quality assurance to only *respond* to problems *after* they have occurred. Prospective quality assurance enables your board and hospital to *prevent* problems, which is the distinction between *building* quality in (prospective quality), and *inspecting* quality in (retrospective quality). It is much better from a cost perspective as well as a quality perspective to focus on building quality into your hospital's care than it is to focus on inspecting quality after the care has been delivered or the new venture or service established.

The prospective approach to quality, that is, reviewing new types of care before they are implemented, is so important that it should be used by your board routinely. In fact, if your board requires a quality plan in all its decisions that in any way affect patient care, it will send a resounding message throughout the hospital that quality is a top priority of the board and of the hospital. This will help ensure that potential quality problems are identified and prevented before they have a negative impact on the quality of patient care. The prospective approach to quality is important, powerful, and uniquely in the board's domain (Orlikoff, 1989).

Understanding Quality Assurance

By this point you should have a fairly firm foundation on the basics of quality in hospitals. From this foundation you and your board will be able to confidently consider many quality and quality-related issues. This foundation will also support your learning other concepts related to quality in your hospital, such as quality assurance.

Quality assurance is defined as the evaluation of patient care, and factors that affect that care, toward the goal of continually improving the quality of that care. This means that there are two general components to quality assurance (Orlikoff, 1990, p. 49):

- *The problem-focused approach:* Those activities designed to eliminate or minimize problems in patient care or bad outcomes of care
- *The continuous quality improvement approach:* those activities designed to make "good" or acceptable (that is, problem-free) patient care even better

Both approaches should be employed by your hospital's quality assurance or quality improvement program. The issue is how to determine the relative emphasis that is placed on each of these important tools.

For example, assume that for some reason your hospital's quality assurance or improvement program could focus on only one of the two general components of quality assurance. It could focus entirely on identifying and resolving problems affecting patient care, or it could focus entirely on making good care better—the continuous quality improvement approach. Which would you choose?

Most trustees choose the continuous quality improvement approach. They do so under the assumption that, in addition to making "good" ("problem-free") care better, this approach will also identify and resolve problems that affect patient care. Although this is a reasonable assumption, it is frequently *not* the case in many hospital quality assurance programs.

One reason for the lack of effective continuous quality improvement is the negative view of quality assurance as a "witch-hunt" (discussed earlier in this chapter). This perspective can actually motivate medical and hospital staff members to *avoid* identifying and resolving problems in patient care, especially if these problems may be caused by or involve other members of the medical or hospital staff. Thus the quality assurance mechanisms that should identify problems in care can be manipulated such that they identify *no* problems. They can also be manipulated so that the only problems identified will be small ones, whereas the significant ones are left unaddressed. This may sound like a farfetched notion, but unfortunately it is quite common in hospitals throughout the country.

Thus a complete focus on the "making good care better" approach may enable the individuals involved in your hospital's quality assessment and improvement activities to actually *avoid* the identification and resolution of problems in patient care. In essence, this can occur when the resources of the quality assurance program are devoted to studying and improving good or acceptable care, while problem areas in care continue without examination or corrective action.

This is not to suggest that the continuous quality improvement approach should not be used in your hospital's quality assurance and improvement program. Instead, the point of this section is to convince you and your fellow trustees that the problem-focused approach of quality assurance should not be abandoned. Why? Very simply, because in all probability your hospital has problems that negatively affect patient care and in some cases actually cause patient injuries. This issue will be discussed in greater detail in chapter 5 under "Risk Management."

The concept of continuous quality improvement, or total quality management, is discussed at length in chapter 9. You and your board need to be aware of what percentage of your quality assurance program's resources and time should be devoted to the problem-focused approach, and what percentage to the continuous quality improvement approach. Generally these relative percentages will vary from hospital to hospital depending on the frequency and seriousness of the quality-related problems. If your hospital has quality-related problems that are not being identified and resolved by any of the many quality assurance activities, then your board should increase the emphasis of the quality assurance program on the problem-focused approach.

A good rule of thumb is to focus a majority of the quality assurance program on the problem-focused approach, say 60 percent or 70 percent, until it can be clearly and objectively demonstrated to the board that there are no quality-related problems in your hospital (this will never happen, however), or that their number and seriousness are well under control.

Your hospital board may decide to implement an entirely different ratio of allocating quality assurance resources, say 70 percent to continuous quality improvement and 30 percent to a problem-focused approach. This is fine as long as the determination is made based on your specific hospital's circumstances. In fact, your board *should* develop its own ratio and direction for the quality assurance and improvement program.

Notice the significance of your board's addressing this issue. Now, your board will actually be *directing* the activities and focus of the quality assurance and improvement program, as opposed to *being directed by it*. Most boards just receive quality assurance information without knowing what it means or why it is being done. These boards are not directing their quality assurance and improvement programs, but are being directed by them; at best they can respond only to the information they receive. These boards rarely have any way of knowing if the information they receive is meaningful. Consequently, they are not exercising effective oversight of their hospital's quality of care or its quality assurance and improvement program.

The Problem-Focused Process

Simply directing your hospital's quality assurance and improvement activities to allocate a certain percentage of their energies and resources to the problem-focused process, however, is not enough. Your board must make certain that the process is functioning effectively.

In order to do this, you and your board must know the steps of the problem-focused process, as well as where the process tends to break down. The problem-focused process consists of five steps:

1. Identifying the problem
2. Assessing the problem (activities that determine the cause and scope of the problem)
3. Implementing corrective action (fixing the problem)
4. Monitoring the results of the corrective action to verify that the problem has been eliminated or reduced to an acceptable degree, and that these results are sustained
5. Documenting the process and following up as appropriate

You have probably used this process, consciously or subconsciously, in your business or at home. In the hospital, however, the process frequently breaks down, commonly between step 2, assessing the problem and step 3, implementing corrective action. It is fairly easy to identify problems, and even to assess them. Once a problem is assessed, the corrective action strategy should be clear and easy to implement. Unfortunately, this does not always happen.

Often after a problem in patient care is identified and assessed, no corrective action will be implemented. This can occur for several reasons. One reason is that the logical or assumed corrective action may be threatening to the physicians and staff involved in the problem. Examples of corrective action may include counseling a practitioner to change his or her behavior, taking disciplinary measures, or, in an extreme case, restricting a practitioner's privileges.

Another reason corrective action may not be implemented is that it may require a change in systems or procedures that is beyond the scope and control of those involved in the problem-focused process. If people do not report this situation to higher levels in the organization where such action would be appropriate, the situation can often get lost in the cracks. Or, conversely, even if the situation is reported to the higher organizational authority, no action may be taken for political, financial, or personal reasons.

Still another reason that blocks the implementation of corrective action is the frequent belief of those involved in the problem-focused process that they have not yet really assessed the problem, when in fact they have; the cause and the scope of the problem are clear, but not to them. Another inhibitor of solving identified and assessed problems is when those involved in the problem-solving process do not have access to the resources necessary to implement the corrective action.

There are many personal, political, financial, and organizational reasons why the problem-solving process frequently breaks down. The result often is that a particular problem will be identified, assessed, then assessed again and again, then dropped from the attention of the committee or group that was investigating the problem. Large amounts of time, attention, and money have been spent on the problem, but the problem still exists and in fact has not been improved at all.

When this happens, the quality assurance process is functioning (just look at all the flurry of activity), but *not functioning effectively.* After all, the point of this process is to *solve* problems, not study them to death. Unfortunately, this is an all-too-common scenario throughout many hospitals. It is unfortunate because it looks as if the quality assurance process is working, and it is "working"; it's just not working correctly—it is not accomplishing anything. It is not improving the quality of care by eliminating or reducing problems in that care; it is allowing those problems to exist, and even allowing new problems to appear.

Do you and your board know how well the problem-focused quality assurance process is functioning in your hospital? Do you know which departments and areas in the hospital are effective quality problem solvers and which are not? Most boards do not know because they do not know how to evaluate whether the process is working.

Knowledge of how to evaluate the effectiveness of quality assurance is the benefit of a board's knowing the problem-focused process. Like the vast majority of quality assurance systems and techniques, the board does not *do* the problem-focused process; it makes certain that it is being done correctly in the hospital. To make this determination, it is necessary to know the simple five steps of the process.

The problem-focused process for evaluating quality assurance is very useful to boards in two ways. First, it serves as a format for presenting summary information to the board. For example, the board could receive a report that showed how many problems were identified last quarter by several medical departments, how many were assessed, how many were corrected, how many were monitored, and so on. Here, the board is not involving itself in specific problems; rather, it is monitoring the effectiveness of the problem-focused process. The board will then know which departments and areas in the hospital are effective problem solvers, and can recognize them as such. The board will also know which departments and areas need assistance or direction in effectively solving quality-related problems.

The problem-focused process can be very useful to your board in another important way; that is, in those rare and sensitive occasions when a specific quality-related problem comes to the board for its attention and action. These are precisely the situations that make most trustees uncomfortable, as the problem will often involve medical issues and physicians, and the trustees are usually laymen. Thus the trustees may not really understand the problem, or they may not wish to argue with physicians who maintain that it is really not a problem or that it is not the business of the board.

In these situations, the board should use the problem-focused process to analyze the problem. The board simply can do this by asking questions such as: How was the problem identified? What were the results of the problem assessment, in other words, what is the cause and scope of the problem? Was corrective action implemented? If so, what action? If not, why not? If action was implemented, did the results solve the problem?

The answers to these questions will enable your board to determine whether the problem-focused process was fully and completely conducted, and whether the process is being blocked from proceeding to the next logical step. Thus after asking such questions your board will be able to address the situation more effectively and confidently.

Further, your board will be able to take action where appropriate. Such action will usually relate to completing the problem-focused process. For example, the board might say to the people involved in the problem, "It is clear that you have identified the problem and that you know its cause and scope. So it is now time to implement corrective action, not to study the problem further."

The last step of the process, documenting the process and following up as appropriate, simply involves clear documentation of the application and results of the previous four steps of the process. This step allows the board, as well as external regulators, to verify that the process is working by tracking its component parts.

Although the problem-focused quality assurance process is no longer emphasized by the Joint Commission on Accreditation of Healthcare Organizations (they now require the "monitoring and evaluation process," which is discussed in the next chapter), it is still a very useful tool for the board. It can help your board evaluate the effectiveness of the overall problem-solving activities of your hospital's quality assurance and quality improvement program. It can also facilitate your board's allocation of resources regarding quality. In addition, it can provide your board with an effective framework for addressing and acting on individual quality-related problems that come to the attention of the board.

It is well worth it for you and your board to learn, become comfortable with, and use the problem-focused process. By doing so your board can more effectively and appropriately oversee both the quality of care of your hospital as well as the effectiveness of your hospital's quality assurance and improvement program.

Conclusion

Why does your hospital do quality assurance? This may seem like an odd question to ask, especially at the end of a chapter on quality and quality assurance. Yet it is absolutely critical for you and your board to firmly answer this question for your hospital.

In response you may answer, "Well, obviously to improve the quality of care we provide." That is the right answer, but is it really the reason that your hospital does quality assurance? Unfortunately, that is *not* the reason that many hospitals do quality assurance.

A large number of hospital chief executive officers, senior managers, medical staff members and leaders, quality assurance professionals, and hospital staff believe that the primary (if not the only) purpose of quality assurance is to gain and maintain accreditation of their hospital from the Joint Commission on Accreditation of Healthcare Organizations. In addition, they might feel that quality assurance is also necessary to meet legal, legislative, and regulatory requirements.

This is a common perspective that severely inhibits quality assurance programs from actually improving the quality of care. This perspective creates a defensive approach to quality that pervades all areas of the hospital. Having a defensive approach to quality means that the leaders and staff of the hospital are motivated to do quality assurance and improvement activities solely to satisfy external agencies. This in turn means that those in the hospital *will do only the minimum quality assurance and improvement activities necessary to satisfy the regulatory requirements*, and they will do them halfheartedly at that. Once those requirements are satisfied, quality assurance loses support and commitment, and its activities dramatically decline. This happens because the "goal" of quality assurance supposedly has been attained, that is, the hospital passed its survey and received accreditation.

Ironically, one of the things that makes a defensive approach to quality a self-defeating activity is that the regulators soon become well aware that the hospitals are doing only enough to get by in quality assurance and improvement. So the regulators change the standards and requirements, making them tougher to force the hospitals to do more effective quality assurance and to develop an honest commitment to it. As you can guess, this only further fuels the fires of defensive quality.

An honest commitment to providing quality care and continuously striving to improve the quality of care can never be regulated or legislated from outside the hospital; it must come from within the hospital, from the board.

If any group can do it, the hospital board must transcend the perilous perspective of defensive quality. It is a perspective that is limited and limiting, that actually *works against* your hospital's improving the quality of care that it provides.

Your board should give serious consideration to this issue, discuss it, and determine what the motivation for quality and quality assurance is in the hospital. Once the board firmly answers the question of why the hospital does quality assurance and quality improvement, why it is interested in and committed to quality, it must make certain that this message is communicated relentlessly throughout the hospital until it becomes so ingrained that the hospital has a culture that supports quality care.

The pure and simple purpose of quality assurance and quality improvement activities is to improve the quality of patient care. Why does *your* hospital do quality assurance?

☐ *References*

Donabedian, A. *Explorations in Quality Assessment and Monitoring,* Vol. 1, *The Definition of Quality and Approaches to Its Assessment.* Ann Arbor, MI: Health Administration Press, 1980.

Longo, D. R., Ciccone, K. R., and Lord, J. T. *Integrated Quality Assessment: A Model for Concurrent Review.* Chicago: American Hospital Publishing, 1989.

Orlikoff, J. E. *Quality from the Top: Working with Hospital Governing Boards to Assure Quality Care—A Guide for Quality Assurance Professionals.* Chicago: Pluribus Press, 1990.

Orlikoff, J. E. Do's and don'ts for quality oversight. *Trustee* 42(3):21, Mar. 1989.

Chapter 5

Effectively Overseeing Quality and Quality Assurance

Introduction

For a board to effectively oversee the quality of care, the quality assurance program, and the quality improvement activities of its hospital, it must be composed of board members who are comfortable with the components of quality and quality assurance. Hopefully, the last chapter made you more comfortable with some of the basic issues of quality and quality assurance.

There are, of course, many other issues and components that relate to quality of care and its improvement. To effectively oversee its hospital's quality of care, quality assurance activities, and medical staff activities, a board must be familiar with the sources of information about the quality of care in its hospital and know how to analyze and act on that information appropriately. The remainder of this book will address these issues. This chapter provides an overview of the other quality-related activities and sources of information within your hospital.

The Hospital Quality Assurance Program

The last chapter addressed the definition and purposes of quality assurance as a concept and as an approach in your hospital. Approaches and activities relating to assessing and improving the quality of care in your hospital are probably included under a formal organizational umbrella called the Quality Assurance (QA) Program. Your hospital may call it by another name, such as the Quality Improvement Program, the Quality Management Program, the Hospitalwide Quality Assurance Program, the Continuous Quality Improvement Program, or the Integrated Quality

Assessment Program. For the sake of brevity, this chapter will use the term *QA Program* (Quality Assurance Program).

Whatever the program is called in your hospital, it is useful for your board to be aware of the goals, organization, components, and scope of the program. This is necessary for your board to be able to periodically determine how effectively the QA Program is functioning. Periodic review of the effectiveness of the QA Program, as well as reallocation of resources and formal action taken to improve the QA Program, is a key function of your board. It is this activity that really helps your board effectively oversee the QA Program without becoming inappropriately overinvolved in the details of the program.

The three best ways for your board to become familiar with and to effectively oversee the organization, approaches, techniques, and effectiveness of your QA Program are to review the QA Plan, to annually reappraise the QA Program, and to regularly meet with the hospital's QA Director (or equivalent). Each of these methods is discussed in this section.

Reviewing the QA Plan

The QA Plan is the document that outlines the purposes, goals, structure, scope, and activities of your hospital's QA Program. Your hospital is required by the Joint Commission (*Accreditation Manual for Hospitals,* 1990) to have a written QA Plan. Unfortunately, many hospitals have a QA Plan for only that reason, not to provide a meaningful road map of the QA Program.

A good QA Plan serves to keep the program focused and on track. Further, a good QA Plan provides a useful reference point to evaluate the effectiveness of the QA Program, to identify its strengths and weaknesses, and to improve the function of the QA Program. This occurs through a comparison of the actual QA Program over the past year to the goals, scope, activities, and functions of the various QA processes and techniques that have been spelled out in the QA Plan. Annual reappraisal of the QA Program, also required by the Joint Commission, should result in modifications and fine-tuning to both the QA Program and the QA Plan. In this way, your hospital's QA Program should always evolve, always improve.

It does not always happen that way, however. If annual reappraisal of your hospital's QA Program is done simply to satisfy Joint Commission requirements (remember the dangers of defensive quality discussed in the last chapter), then it may very well have no real positive impact whatsoever on the QA Program. If, however, reappraisal of the QA Program is conducted sincerely and with commitment, then it will most likely result in continuous improvement in the QA Program, and thus in continuous improvement in your hospital's quality of care. As you might guess, your board can play a decisive role in the sincerity, commitment, and resulting effectiveness of the annual reappraisal of the QA Program.

The first step necessary for your board to ensure an effective reappraisal is to review your hospital's QA Plan. This document should do more than simply broadly spell out the purposes, goals, structure, and functions of the QA Program and related activities. The QA Plan should also contain information such as how your hospital defines quality and the level of commitment your hospital has to quality and quality assurance. Further, the QA Plan should also spell out the relative roles of the board, management, medical staff, and nursing and hospital staff regarding the QA Program. It should also clearly define the role of the QA Director (or equivalent), and that of all quality assurance committees.

Most important, your QA Plan should be a working document. That is, it should state *what* activities will be done, *when* they will be performed, *who* will perform them, and *how and when* information from these activities will be communicated throughout the organization (for example, how frequently and in what format information will be communicated to the board). In this way, the QA Plan will contain enough information to easily allow your board to use the QA Plan to annually assess the effectiveness of the QA Program.

Reappraising the QA Program

In its *Guide to Quality Assurance,* (1988, p. 45), the Joint Commission states that annual reappraisal of the QA Program should include:

- Assessment of the monitoring and evaluation process to determine its effectiveness (this process is reviewed in the next section of this chapter)
- Comparison of the written plan with the quality assurance activities that were performed
- Determination of whether quality assurance information was communicated accurately and to the appropriate persons, committees, or other groups
- Determination of whether identified problems were resolved and patient care was improved

An excellent way for your board to exercise effective governance oversight of the QA Program is to meaningfully and actively participate in the annual reappraisal of the QA Program. Your board should assess the QA Program to verify that four crucial objectives have been achieved. These four objectives are as follows:

- *The QA Program has indeed been hospitalwide.* This simply means that all areas, services, and departments of the hospital have meaningfully participated in organized quality assurance activities. Further, it means that *all* individuals in the hospital who provide care to or interact with patients (physicians, nurses, therapists, lab technicians, social services professionals, and so forth) routinely have their care evaluated and their performance reviewed. The failure of hospital QA Programs to be hospitalwide and review all health care providers' care has been the root cause of many serious and preventable patient injuries and the malpractice cases and large losses they in turn generated.

- *The QA Program has identified and resolved problems in patient care.* Remember the discussion of the problem-focused process in chapter 4? If your board, in conjunction with the hospital's QA Director and medical staff leadership, determined that the QA Program should have a specific target for the relative percentage of quality assurance activities devoted to identifying and resolving problems, now is the time to determine whether that target was met. Your board should, however, make certain that these problem-focused activities were *effective* in resolving problems and monitoring them to verify that they remain resolved. Your board should make certain that the QA Program and related activities did not just primarily identify and assess problems.

- *The QA Program has been integrated with other quality-related activities in the hospital.* Many hospital QA Programs and related activities can be described as a "headless octopus." That is, there is a lot of activity, care is being reviewed, studies are being done (the tentacles of the octopus); but nothing is being done with the information generated by this activity. The information does not flow to a central group—the board or a committee—who makes certain that the information is integrated and *used appropriately* (the head of the octopus). Other quality-related activities that frequently are not integrated with the QA Program include medical staff appointments and privilege delineations, infection control, risk management, safety and security programs, and patient representative programs. These issues are discussed in this chapter, except medical staff appointments and privilege delineations, which are reviewed in depth in chapter 6. Your board should assess the program to verify that information is flowing among these activities, that the information is being used, that there is a head on the octopus (a central coordinating function), and that duplication of effort is kept to a minimum.

- *The QA Program has improved the quality of care.* This last point should be the real purpose of annual reappraisal of the QA Program. As mentioned in the last chapter, the *real* purpose of your QA Program should be *to improve the quality of patient care.* Thus annual reappraisal of the QA Program should focus on this issue. Did your QA Program improve the quality of care in your hospital last year? This is the bottom-line issue.

If your QA Program did in fact improve the quality of patient care, how and where did it do so? Do not just take someone's word that care is better. If the care is in fact better, it can and should be demonstrated to the board (this is why it is important to develop a definition of quality that is measurable). If it cannot be demonstrated to the board, that is a good indication that the care has not in fact been improved. If the quality of care did not improve, why did it not? How can the QA Program be strengthened so it is more effective in improving the quality of care in the coming year? What action should the board take to facilitate this? These are the questions you should ask yourself about your QA Program. They are also the questions your board should ask as it participates in annual reappraisal of the QA Program.

Meeting with the QA Professional

The last portion of this section is devoted to an individual in your hospital who is, or should be, a key player in your hospital's QA Program and quality of care: the QA professional or QA director. This is the hospital staff person who has responsibility for the QA Program and related activities.

Most QA professionals are not really used to their full potential to improve the hospital's quality of care because most hospitals take an externally motivated, defensive approach to quality. Thus the time and efforts of most QA professionals is largely spent crunching numbers, churning out data, and generating meeting minutes and other massive quantities of paper. This is done to *satisfy the Joint Commission and other regulators, not to improve the quality of care.*

Unfortunately, the defensive approach to quality occurs at a time when many hospitals are broadcasting, both internally and externally, their "commitment to quality." If your hospital is really committed to quality, your QA professional should see that commitment in terms of financial and organizational support for the QA Program and related activities. Many hear about it, but they do not see such commitment and as a result are becoming very demoralized. As you assess your hospital's commitment to quality consider this: your hospital may have a chief financial officer or equivalent who is at the vice-president level. At what level of the organization is the QA professional? Does your hospital have a chief quality officer or equivalent? This is not to say that you should rally your board to create such a position. Instead, you and your board should honestly assess and, if appropriate, upgrade your hospital's true commitment to quality and the QA Program. This will often involve upgrading your commitment to the hospital's QA professional.

Meetings between your board and the QA professional will help you really assess your hospital's commitment to quality. The QA professional can also be instrumental in orienting your board to the specifics of your QA Program and in presenting quality assurance and quality-related information to the board. The QA professional can either be a low-level number cruncher whose primary job is to make certain that the requirements of the Joint Commission and other regulators are met, or this person can be the spearhead of the QA Program and quality improvement efforts and a quality consultant to the board. The choice is up to your board.

The Monitoring and Evaluation Process

As was mentioned in chapter 4, the Joint Commission no longer emphasizes the problem-focused process in quality assurance activities. This, however, does not mean that it is not a useful tool for boards. Instead of the problem-focused process, the Joint Commission now requires that hospital quality assurance activities employ a 10-step monitoring and evaluation process.

The Joint Commission calls the monitoring and evaluation process "the cornerstone of effective quality assurance activities," and so you should have a passing familiarity with it. The Joint Commission's monitoring and evaluation process (*Guide to Quality Assurance*, 1988, p. 51) consists of the following steps:

1. Assign responsibility for monitoring and evaluation activities.
2. Delineate scope of care [to be monitored].
3. Identify important aspects of care [high-risk, high-volume or aspects prone to problems].
4. Identify indicators [of quality related to those aspects of care; an indicator is a well-defined, measurable variable related to the structure, process, or outcome of care].
5. Establish thresholds for evaluation [the level or point at which intensive evaluation of care is triggered; a threshold should be established for each indicator].
6. Collect and organize data.
7. Evaluate care. [When the cumulative data reach the threshold for evaluation, appropriate staff members should evaluate the care provided to determine whether a problem exists.]

8. Take actions to solve problems.
9. Assess the actions and document improvement.
10. Communicate relevant information to the organizationwide quality assurance program.

Clearly, the monitoring and evaluation process is an expanded version of the problem-focused process discussed in chapter 4. Extensive knowledge of the monitoring and evaluation process is certainly required for those "in the trenches," those medical and hospital staff members who are actually doing quality assurance. It is not necessary, however, that you or members of your board become experts in this process, or even track it closely. Instead, the board should monitor the hospital quality assurance activities to verify that the monitoring and evaluation process is in place throughout the hospital and functioning effectively. This can be accomplished most easily by the board through use of the problem-focused process.

If the monitoring and evaluation process is functioning effectively, it will identify problems in, or opportunities to improve, the quality of care and assess those problems and develop and implement action to improve the care or reduce the problems. Thus if the 10-step monitoring and evaluation process is functioning, it will be evident in the successful progression through the five steps of the problem-focused process.

The monitoring and evaluation process may be useful background for you and other members of the board, but there is no need to commit it to memory. The monitoring and evaluation process is a necessary and useful tool for those medical and hospital staff actually *conducting* quality assurance activities. The problem-focused process, however, represents a more appropriate *governance* tool for your board to assess the effectiveness of quality assurance processes and to address individual problems that come to the attention of the board.

Clinical Quality Reviews and Information

There is an old joke among quality assurance professionals, that the patient's medical record gets more attention than the patient. This refers to the large number of reviews that the Joint Commission requires be performed when certain types of care are provided or certain procedures are performed. For example, did you know that in your hospital the following events and activities are supposed to be reviewed: every single surgical procedure, every death, every time blood or blood components are given to a patient, every time certain drugs and antibiotics are given to patients? Many of these routine reviews and monitoring activities of the medical staff are conducted using the monitoring and evaluation process.

As indicated earlier, the problem with many of these reviews is that they are conducted simply to satisfy external requirements. Consequently, the reviews are performed often but not well, that is, they fail to identify negative trends or problems, or they identify them but justify them as "acceptable and expected complications of care." Alternatively, they may identify problems but fail to take corrective action.

It is not necessary (or wise) for your board to spend its time routinely assessing the results of these reviews. Instead, the board should periodically receive information that indicates whether these reviews are functioning effectively, are identifying and resolving problems, and are being integrated into other quality-related activities such as medical staff credentialing (appointments to the medical staff and the delineation of privileges).

Clinical quality reviews can and should be generating extremely useful information for the QA Program, the medical staff credentialing functions, and your hospital's overall efforts to improve quality of care. If they are not, that is a good indication that your hospital is playing the defensive quality game. If these reviews are not functioning effectively in your hospital, it is appropriate for your board to turn its attention to this issue and take action to improve the effectiveness of the reviews. Such action may include informing those individuals responsible for the reviews that they are being performed inappropriately and requesting explanations, directing corrective action, directing more resources to support the reviews, bringing in external consultants to assess and improve the reviews, and many others.

Such action will of course involve interacting with the medical staff and may therefore be politically sensitive and intimidating to you or some fellow board members. Nevertheless, it is your board's responsibility to direct the resources of your hospital to correct such problems in the QA Program when they become apparent. If your board neglects to take action, it is then contributing to the defensive quality perspective and ineffectiveness of the QA Program.

Infection Control

One of the quality assurance–related activities of your hospital is infection control. Infection control relates to the identification and control of infections that are caused by and that occur in the hospital. Your hospital's Infection Control Program may be formally organized under your QA Program, such that the professional responsible for infection control reports to the person responsible for quality assurance (or it may be organized differently). Regardless of the organizational relationship of infection control to quality assurance, your board should be aware of the extremely important function of infection control and of the seriousness of infections in hospitals.

Nosocomial (hospital-acquired) infections are a very serious threat in hospitals and have significant implications for both the cost and quality of care. Consider these grim statistics:

- There are at least 100,000 nosocomial infection–related deaths per year in the United States (Nahata, 1985).
- A *minimum* of 5 to 6 percent of all patients in acute care general hospitals sustain nosocomial infections. This generates nosocomial infections in somewhere between 1.5 to 2.1 million patients every year. The deaths caused by these infections put nosocomial infections in the top 10 causes of deaths in this country (Joint Commission on Accreditation of Healthcare Organizations, 1988, p. 126; Haley and others, 1987, p. 1611).
- The average nosocomial infection *that does not result in death* increases the patient's length of stay in the hospital by four days and costs the hospital about $1,800 (Holzman, 1988).
- Infection is the most frequent cause of death in cancer patients (Inlander and others, 1988, p.124; Elting and others, 1986).
- The aggregate cost of nosocomial infections in the United States is somewhere between $2 billion and $4 billion (Haley and others, 1987, p. 1611; Missouri Professional Liability Insurance Association, 1978).

Unfortunately, the already-serious problem of nosocomial infections may become worse in the future. This is due to many variables, some of which can be controlled by the hospital, others of which cannot. Variables that will contribute to the increasing incidence of nosocomial infections include nursing and staff shortages within the hospital; the development of more antibiotic-resistant organisms that generate infections; the increased use of invasive procedures; more immunologically suppressed patients—such as those with AIDS, who are more prone to nosocomial infections; and the growing elderly population, who are also more prone to nosocomial infections (Longo and others, 1988, p. 75).

Nosocomial infections are caused by a myriad of factors within the hospital, many of which involve human error. According to Inlander and others (1988, p. 128), some of the most common causes of nosocomial infections in the hospital are:

- Lack of hand washing by medical and hospital staff
- Poor personal hygiene
- Faulty patient care technique
- Improper sterilization or disinfection of reusable items (surgical instruments, bedpans, thermometers)

- Inadequate refrigeration of food (the leading cause of nosocomial outbreaks of salmonellosis)
- Inadequate cooking and reheating of food

Nosocomial infections can be classified in several ways—by the organism causing the infection, the body part that sustained the initial infection, or the area of the hospital where the infection occurred. It is useful to know what the most common types of nosocomial infection are in your hospital so that your board can make certain that infection control efforts are optimally focused.

One of the most common types of nosocomial infection is urinary tract infection caused by the use of urinary catheters. On average for all hospitals, urinary tract infections account for about 42 percent of all nosocomial infections, followed by (in descending order) surgical wound infections, 24 percent; pneumonia, 10 percent; bacteremia, 5 percent; and all other infections, 19 percent (Haley and others, 1985).

Clearly, nosocomial infections can have an impact on the overall quality of care your hospital provides. Consequently it is important for your board to be aware of the nosocomial infection situation in your hospital, as well as the effectiveness of your Infection Control Program. Your board should monitor the Infection Control Program to make certain that it has sufficient resources and is functioning effectively to track as well as *prevent and reduce* the incidence of nosocomial infections. Further, your board should monitor to ensure that the Infection Control Program is operating on a concurrent basis and is closely integrated with the QA Program.

For starters, here are some questions you and your board should be able to answer regarding nosocomial infections and the Infection Control Program in your hospital. What was the nosocomial infection rate for your hospital for the past 12 months? Is that higher or lower than the preceding 12 months? Is the nosocomial infection rate trend (by month or by quarter) going up or down in your hospital? Are there any areas in your hospital that consistently demonstrate higher-than-average nosocomial infection rates? What positive steps are being taken to prevent and reduce nosocomial infections? Are they effective?

Asking these questions of your hospital management, QA Professional, or Infection Control Coordinator is an appropriate and necessary first step for you and your board to learn about nosocomial infection control in your hospital. It is also the first step toward effective board oversight of, and commitment to, this critically important quality-related function.

Risk Management

Do you know that hospitals can be dangerous places that actually *cause injuries* to patients? More specifically, do you know what areas in your hospital pose the greatest risk of injuries to patients? These and other questions raise the important quality-related function of risk management.

Risk management involves those activities that identify areas of potential injury to patients in your hospital, that minimize the chances those injuries will occur, and that attempt to reduce risk of malpractice claims and losses those injuries can generate. Risk management also involves the broader activities of malpractice and general liability insurance purchasing and claims management (handling allegations of malpractice *after* claims are filed).

The primary focus of risk management in your hospital should be on the *prevention* of injuries and of malpractice claims and losses, not on how to respond to them *after* they occur. Thus the patient-injury prevention focus of risk management should closely link the function of risk management with the QA Program and medical staff credentialing activities in your hospital. This is such an important issue, one that directly relates to quality, that your board should receive regular reports on risk management and monitor the program to ensure it is functioning effectively. Following are some guidelines on how your board can effectively oversee your hospital's Risk Management Program.

Evaluating Risk Management Priorities

Your board must first understand that there are two broad categories of injuries that can occur in, and be caused by, your hospital: custodial-related injury and iatrogenic injury (Orlikoff and Vanagunas, 1988, p. 39).

Custodial-related injuries are those not specifically related to or caused by physicians or other professional health care providers in your hospital. Instead, they are caused by administrative or custodial actions, inactions, or circumstances. Examples of custodial-related injuries that frequently occur in hospitals are patient falls from bed; falls in or on the way to the bathroom; slips and falls on wet or waxed floors; slips and falls caused by clutter in hallways, driveways, parking lots, or by poor lighting in any of those areas; cuts, bruises, or burns from improperly operated or faulty equipment; and the like. Custodial injuries are often referred to as slips-and-falls injuries. Basically, custodial-related injury is not specific to a hospital but can occur most anywhere, such as in a hotel.

Iatrogenic injuries, on the other hand, can occur *only* in a hospital or under the care of a physician or other health care provider. Iatrogenic injuries are *medically related injuries*, those caused by or directly related to the actions (or inactions) of physicians or other professional health care providers.

Examples of typical iatrogenic injuries include most nosocomial infections; a surgical procedure performed on the wrong body part, or removal of the wrong body organ (yes, this does happen); a surgical procedure performed on the wrong patient; damage caused to a patient's colon during a colonoscopy (an invasive procedure that involves inserting a tube into a patient's colon that allows a physician to visually examine the colon); misdiagnosis of a patient's condition; a patient's allergic reaction to a prescribed drug (serious allergic reactions are referred to as "anaphylactic" reactions and can result in death); and many others. (Taken in this context, Hammurabi's definition of quality was really the absence of specific iatrogenic injuries.)

Another difference between custodial and iatrogenic injuries relates to *how* injuries are measured and defined. There are two ways to measure hospital injuries that occur in patients, family members, visitors, and staff. Injuries can be measured by their *frequency,* how often that type of injury occurs; or they can be measured by their *severity,* the seriousness of the injury in terms of the physical consequences to the patient and the financial consequences (malpractice dollar losses) to the hospital.

Custodial-related injuries are the most *frequently* occurring injuries, accounting for about 75 to 85 percent of all patient injuries. Although custodial injuries occur most frequently, they tend to be much less severe than iatrogenic injuries. Measured in terms of malpractice dollar losses, custodial injuries account for only about 15 to 25 percent of all hospital aggregate malpractice dollar losses (Orlikoff, 1990, pp. 72-73).

Iatrogenic injuries, on the other hand, occur far less frequently than do custodial injuries. When iatrogenic injuries occur, however, they tend to be far more severe and serious than custodial injuries. Iatrogenic injuries account for about 75 to 85 percent of all malpractice dollar losses for hospitals (Orlikoff, 1990, p. 72).

Your hospital's Risk Management Program should address both types of injury. The issue is, where should the majority of the risk management resources be devoted? Let's say that knowing what you now know about the difference between custodial and iatrogenic injuries, your board is presented with a choice. Suppose that your board is told that your Risk Management Program can focus only on preventing and minimizing custodial *or* iatrogenic injuries in your hospital, but not both. Which would you choose? Most trustees answer by saying the Risk Management Program should focus on iatrogenic injuries. This answer makes sense because these are the types of injuries that can cause the most harm to the patient and the most malpractice loss and bad publicity for the hospital.

Clearly, however, your hospital's Risk Management Program should address preventing *both* types of injuries. But which type of injury should be the major priority of the Risk Management Program? Should the program devote a majority of its efforts and resources to custodial or to iatrogenic injuries? Again, you probably picked iatrogenic injuries as the most important focus for your hospital's program (and you would be correct if you did). Now, if that approach is so logically clear, why is it that a majority of hospital Risk Management Programs focus on *custodial* and not *iatrogenic* injuries?

There are several reasons for this unfortunate situation. One is that custodial injuries and events are easier to measure than iatrogenic events. The most important reason, however, is that custodial events are often less threatening to physicians and hospital staff, so they do not mind reporting them. Iatrogenic events, on the other hand, usually involve physicians. Often the physicians may be threatened or offended at the concept that they were involved in or caused an adverse event or injury to a patient. Therefore, they may not report it, or they may put pressure on nurses and other hospital staff to refrain from reporting it.

Which type of injury does *your* Risk Management Program focus on? Is it an appropriate focus, or should it be changed? This is an appropriate question for your board to ask. Do not be surprised if the answer is that your hospital's Risk Management Program focuses on custodial injuries and not sufficiently on iatrogenic injuries. If this is the case, it is time for your board to ask why and to take governance action to redirect the priorities of the Risk Management Program.

Evaluating the Incident Reporting System

One of the major tools of a Risk Management Program is the incident or occurrence report. This is a form used to alert the Risk Manager about an actual or potentially adverse event. The vast majority of hospital incident reports relate to custodial, not iatrogenic, events.

The incident report serves as a concurrent care measurement device that facilitates several activities. First, it should generate an immediate response to the injured patient. Second, it should facilitate an immediate investigation into what caused the incident or occurrence and result in action to prevent the incident or occurrence from happening again, or to minimize the chances that it will occur again. Third, incident reports can be analyzed to *predict which patients may file malpractice claims or lawsuits in the future,* and thus enable a hospital to prepare a defense or to establish sufficient financial reserves.

Does your hospital have an effective incident or occurrence reporting system? Does it focus exclusively or primarily on custodial injuries, or does it focus on iatrogenic injuries? Are incident reports responded to appropriately and quickly? Do they result in corrective action? Finally, do your incident reports accurately predict your malpractice claims?

This last question is an excellent way for your board to assess the effectiveness of the incident reporting system. A simple graph provided to your board once or twice a year that compares incident reports to malpractice claims will tell whether your incident reporting system is adequately predicting malpractice claims and focusing on areas of iatrogenic injuries. (A sample of such a graph is presented in figure 7-7 in chapter 7.)

Addressing High-Risk Areas

What are the areas in your hospital where patients are most likely to be injured iatrogenically? According to national aggregate data, the highest-risk areas of iatrogenic injury in hospitals tend to be the surgical suite, the emergency room, the labor and delivery room(s), special care units (such as intensive care units, cardiac care units, and so forth), and the patient's room (Orlikoff and Vanagunas, 1988, p. 40).

Once your board knows the specific high-risk areas for your hospital, it should make certain that these areas and departments have effective risk management and quality assurance activities devoted to them. Is this the case in your hospital? Does your board monitor the highest-risk areas to make certain that they actively participate in effective risk management and quality assurance activities? These are some of the ways that your board can take an active, yet appropriate, governance role in minimizing the risk of serious patient injury and improving the quality of care in your hospital.

Information on Patient Satisfaction

As discussed earlier, one aspect by which your hospital may define quality is the perspective of its patients. Thus it is appropriate for your board to receive periodic reports that indicate the level of patient satisfaction with your hospital.

Your hospital may use several different systems to gather information from patients. These may include patient complaint-gathering and assessment mechanisms, patient surveys upon discharge from the hospital, postdischarge surveys, or special polls or focused surveys of patients in particular areas (such as the high-risk areas discussed in the previous section). In addition to, or in support of, these activities, your hospital may have a Guest Relations Program, a patient representative, or some other person or area that performs this function.

Regardless of which of these functions or programs your hospital has (and it *should* have at least a Patient Complaint Program), it is important that your board be aware of the activity. Even more important is the need for your board to receive periodic reports from these activities or programs. In response to these reports your board should ask questions and, depending on the answers, take action.

Examples of important questions are:

- Does our hospital have an effective patient complaint collection and response mechanism?
- Which are the areas of our hospital that generate the most patient complaints?
- What is the hospital's response to these areas of highest complaint? Is the response working? If not, what else is being done?
- What are the areas that generate the *least* number of patient complaints? How is the hospital responding to these areas? Are they being recognized and rewarded?

Paying attention to the perspective of the patients of your hospital is an important way for your board to track and oversee this important perspective of quality care. Patient satisfaction information can thus be extremely valuable governance information and can enable your board to direct appropriate action when necessary to maintain or improve this key aspect of your hospital's quality of care.

Staff Perspectives and Information

Another important perspective on quality is that of the hospital staff. Their perceptions about the strengths and weaknesses of the hospital's quality care are often on target and thus valuable to the hospital's quality assurance and quality improvement efforts.

Therefore, your board should make certain that mechanisms exist in your hospital to candidly and accurately assess the perspectives of your staff. These mechanisms may include staff surveys, staff complaint collection and response programs, and staff suggestion programs. More expansively, Continuous Quality Improvement Programs or Total Quality Management Programs (discussed in detail in chapter 9) are based on staff perceptions, involvement, and empowerment.

Your board should make certain that the most important resource of your hospital, its people, are involved in improving the quality of care they provide. This transcends their participation in quality assurance and quality-related activities, and focuses more on their feelings and perceptions about the levels of quality in the hospital and what can be done to improve them. Does your board monitor the perceptions of the medical staff, hospital staff, and employees? Are you taking advantage of your hospital's most important resource?

Quality-Related Information from Outside the Hospital

The vast majority of the material in this chapter and in chapter 4 addressed quality-related information that comes from *inside* your hospital. For reasons discussed earlier, it is absolutely critical that your board ensure that your hospital maintains an internally motivated focus on quality. This means that your board and hospital should place a priority on quality-related information that is generated within the hospital.

As stated earlier, some factors that motivate a *defensive quality* approach are *externally imposed* requirements relating to quality. Another factor is the external information about your hospital's quality of care that your hospital may be obligated to respond to.

Although your hospital's QA Program and quality improvement efforts should not be *driven* by external requirements and information, this information can be useful as *one component* of the information it analyzes to assess and improve quality. Thus your board should understand the external information that may be useful to your internally driven QA Program and quality improvement efforts. This type of information, presented to your board in the proper perspective, can enhance your board's understanding and effective oversight of your hospital's quality of care. This external information includes:

- *Results of Joint Commission on Accreditation of Healthcare Organization surveys:* This information, in addition to relating to achieving and maintaining your hospital's accreditation, is also extremely useful as an external assessment of your hospital's QA Program, quality improvement activities, and effectiveness of medical staff participation in these activities.
- *Professional Review Organization and Health Care Financing Administration actions and data:* If your hospital has received sanctions from your PRO or HCFA, what is the reason for this?
- *Third-party payers:* Increasingly, third-party payers of health care, such as employers and insurance companies, are concerned about the quality of care they are paying for. Some of them compile data on hospital quality and share it with the hospitals they do business with or are considering doing business with.
- *Malpractice insurer information:* Many insurers of hospitals conduct loss-control (risk management) surveys of the hospitals they insure or are planning to insure. These reports are usually shared with the hospitals.

There are many other types of external information about your hospital's quality of care. Your board should receive summary reports of this information and use it in several ways. One valuable way to use it is as an external assessment of your quality assurance and quality improvement activities, to compare your internal assessments with the external assessments, and to address significant differences. Another way to use this information is as yet another (but not the primary) component of defining the quality of care that your hospital provides.

External information about the quality of care can be useful to your board and your hospital in your efforts to constantly assess and improve your quality of care. This information must be taken in its proper perspective, however, to avoid the seductive but specious trap of adopting an externally motivated, defensive approach to quality. A key responsibility of your board is to make certain that your hospital can use this information and address external requirements without losing the crucial internal motivation for quality.

Conclusion

This chapter has presented many sources of information about the quality of care in your hospital. It has also reviewed how your board can use this information to effectively oversee your hospital's quality of care and QA Program in a manner appropriate to the policy/oversight role of your board.

For this information to be meaningful to you as a board member, you must use it. The best way to use it is as the basis for asking for quality-related reports to the board, as a method for evaluating those reports, and, most important, as the basis for asking questions about those reports.

Do not be afraid to ask quality-related questions during board or committee meetings. Whether you ask questions of your hospital chief executive officer, a medical staff leader, or other board members, it is important to remember this tip for trustees: *There is no such thing as a stupid question about quality.*

Many quality-related problems in hospitals were once buried, justified as acceptable, or written off as "a fact of life, a cost of doing business, or something that can't be changed." However, such problems were unearthed, seriously examined, and corrected as a direct result of one little "stupid question" asked by a trustee. Hopefully this chapter has made you a little more confident to ask questions about quality, and a little more knowledgeable about how to respond to the answers.

References

Elting, L. S., Bodey, G. P., and Fainstein, V. Polymicrobial septicemia in the cancer patient. *Medicine* 65(4), July 1986.

Haley, R. W., Culver, D. H., White, J. W., Morgan, W. M., and Emori, T. G. The nationwide nosocomial infection rate. *American Journal of Epidemiology,* Feb. 1985.

Haley, R. W., White, J. W., Culver, D. H., and Hughes, J. M. The financial incentive for hospitals to prevent nosocomial infections under the prospective payment system. *Journal of the American Medical Association,* 257(12):1611–14, Mar. 1987.

Holzman, D. The sickly side of hospital stays. *Insight,* Apr. 18, 1988.

Inlander, C. B., Levin, L. S., and Weiner, E. *Medicine on Trial: The Appalling Story of Medical Ineptitude and the Arrogance that Overlooks It.* New York City: Pantheon Books, 1988.

Joint Commission on Accreditation of Healthcare Organizations. *The Joint Commission Guide to Quality Assurance.* Chicago: JCAHO, 1988.

Joint Commission on Accreditation of Healthcare Organizations. *Accreditation Manual for Hospitals.* Chicago: JCAHO, 1990.

Longo, D. R., Ciccone, K. R., and Lord, J. T. *Integrated Quality Assessment: A Model for Concurrent Review.* Chicago: American Hospital Publishing, 1989.

Missouri Professional Liability Insurance Association. *Risk Management Letter.* Jefferson City, MO: MPLIA, Dec. 1978.

Nahata, M. C. Handwashing prevents infections. *Drug Intelligence and Clinical Pharmacy,* Oct. 1985.

Orlikoff, J. E. *Quality from the Top: Working with Hospital Governing Boards to Assure Quality Care—A Guide for Quality Assurance Professionals.* Chicago: Pluribus Press, 1990.

Orlikoff, J. E., and Vanagunas, A. M. *Malpractice Prevention and Liability Control for Hospitals,* 2d ed. Chicago: American Hospital Publishing, 1988.

Chapter 6

The Board's Role in Medical Staff Credentialing

Introduction

Perhaps the board's most important quality assurance responsibility is the credentialing of the hospital's medical staff. For most hospital boards, this is the most difficult of all the governance functions to perform effectively.

For many hospital trustees, the issue of the board's role in medical staff credentialing causes much anxiety and doubt. "After all," many trustees have said, "how can a board composed of mostly *laymen* decide whether a physician is qualified or competent enough to be on the medical staff?" This issue of why and how a lay board decides which physicians can practice at the hospital and what procedures they can perform is very intimidating to most trustees. It is also an issue that can be very threatening to physicians. Hence the controversial nature of the board's role in medical staff credentialing.

Medical staff credentialing encompasses the policies, procedures, and all activities surrounding the initial appointment and reappointment of physicians (and other health care practitioners, such as dentists) to the hospital's medical staff. Medical staff credentialing also involves granting and renewing of clinical privileges to medical staff members. Basically, then, credentialing involves deciding which physicians may join the medical staff, which physicians may remain on the medical staff, which procedures each physician will be allowed to perform, and which diseases or categories of diseases the physician will be allowed to treat. Although the medical staff *recommends* these credentialing decisions, it is the hospital board that actually *makes* the final decision.

The primary purpose of your hospital's medical staff credentialing system is to ensure that only qualified physicians are granted practice privileges and that physicians practice within the scope of their capabilities and expertise. Because this evaluation is done *prior to* a physician's initial appointment or reappointment, credentialing, when properly conducted, is an excellent example of prospective quality assurance (discussed in chapter 4). Development and use of an appropriate credentialing system is essential if your hospital is to achieve and maintain a desired level of quality care and minimize the risks of medically related patient injury that can result in malpractice losses.

Physicians, as clinical decision-making authorities in the hospital, profoundly affect the hospital's overall level of quality of care. Yet despite physicians' impact on quality and the board's ultimate accountability for physician performance, many boards continue to discharge their credentialing oversight responsibility in an ineffective, outdated, and inappropriate mode. Unfortunately these governing boards merely "rubber stamp" the medical staff's recommendations about who should be a medical staff member and what privileges they should have.

A recent survey on disagreements among hospital governing boards, executives, and medical staffs (Joint Commission on Accreditation of Healthcare Organizations, 1987, p. 7) found that physician credentialing ranked among the top 10 points of conflict among these groups. This finding is not really surprising, given the long history of individual physician responsibility for patient care quality and the board's relatively recent involvement in and accountability for it.

Yet governing boards that choose the rubber stamp approach to credentialing to avoid conflict are exposing themselves and their hospitals to significant potential liability. At the same time, they are missing an important opportunity to strengthen their relationship with the medical staff by collaboratively discharging this critical leadership responsibility.

Hospital boards that are effectively operating in an active oversight mode have trustees who know the board's responsibility and accountability for medical staff credentialing and understand the credentialing process and their role in it. This chapter discusses the board's accountability for medical staff credentialing and describes the roles of the board, medical staff, and hospital executives in effectively conducting the credentialing process. This chapter also suggests a collaborative approach that can be used to help your hospital board make more consistent and objective credentialing decisions on medical staff candidates.

The Board's Expanding Accountability

As mentioned in chapter 3, the landmark case of *Darling v. Charleston Memorial Hospital* was the beginning of a wave of legal cases that further delineated the governing board's ultimate accountability for patient care quality. As chapter 3 also demonstrated, many of these cases focused on the hospital's, and therefore the governing board's, responsibility for physician capability, competence, and performance. Legal cases such as those listed in chapter 3 (and others that your hospital CEO will be able to provide to you) all expand and reinforce the hospital board's ultimate responsibility for patient care quality through the medical staff credentialing function.

In addition to its *quality* implications, credentialing also has *liability* implications for the hospital and its board. A hospital board that oversees a credentialing system that allows incompetent physicians to join or remain on the medical staff, or that allows physicians to practice procedures they are not qualified to practice, increases the risk of medically related patient injury and malpractice liability. On the other hand, a board that condones a credentialing system that unfairly denies medical staff membership or privileges to qualified physicians runs the risk of a physician suing the hospital and board for restraint of trade or antitrust violations. Thus credentialing can be a double-edged sword of liability, with either patients or physicians suing the hospital.

Legal Mandates

Although many legal cases regarding physician credentialing have been decided in favor of the hospital (Orlikoff and Totten, 1988, p. 15), liability has been incurred when governing boards failed to ensure that an appropriate credentialing process exists and was in fact conducted. Hospitals have been found liable when patient injury resulted from lack of appropriate diligence in conducting physician credentialing. Liability also can occur when physicians successfully claim that inappropriate credentialing resulted in economic loss to them through the hospital's antitrust activities, which was the situation in *Patrick v. Burget* (1988).

In this case, Dr. Timothy Patrick, a general and vascular surgeon practicing in Astoria, Oregon, contended that his denial of privileges at Columbia Memorial Hospital, Astoria's only hospital, was motivated by a desire to restrict competition. He claimed that the hospital's peer review activities had been initiated and conducted by physicians who were staff members at the hospital and members of the Astoria Clinic. The clinic was a group practice in which Dr. Patrick had declined to accept partnership, preferring to set up his own practice in competition with it.

After Dr. Patrick established his own practice, the clinic physicians refused to have professional dealings with him, declining to provide consultations or back-up coverage for his patients. At the same time, they criticized him for failing to obtain consultations or coverage and complained about his medical practices to the State Board of Medical

Examiners. Clinic physicians also requested review of Dr. Patrick's hospital privileges. After the hospital's medical staff executive committee voted to terminate Dr. Patrick's privileges, clinic physicians also participated in the hearing he requested to review the termination.

Dr. Patrick filed suit, claiming that the clinic physicians participated in the hospital's peer review activities to reduce competition rather than to improve the quality of patient care. The clinic physicians denied the assertion and the court turned the matter over to a jury, which supported Dr. Patrick's claim. Antitrust damages of approximately $2 million were awarded to Dr. Patrick.

Upon appeal, the circuit court ruled that despite the motivation of the clinic physicians to use peer review to restrict competition, the matter was exempt from federal antitrust scrutiny. The court reasoned that hospital peer review instead fell under the state action doctrine.

The case went to the U.S. Supreme Court, which reversed the appeals court. The Supreme Court found that whereas the state of Oregon had a policy favoring peer review, the state did not actively supervise hospital peer review decisions and, therefore, the state action exemption did not apply. Ultimately, the district court's $2 million judgment in favor of Dr. Patrick was upheld.

It is important that all trustees on your board understand that the hospital's accountability and liability for the credentialing function exist primarily to protect patients as well as to ensure fair, thorough, and consistent consideration of physician requests for privileges. Trustees must ensure that their credentialing process is thorough, fair, and free from conflicts of interest such as those that existed in the *Patrick* case.

Legislative Mandates

In addition to a body of legal cases that clearly demonstrates board accountability for medical staff credentialing, the 1986 Health Care Quality Improvement Act also focuses squarely on hospital requirements for participation in the credentialing process. The act provides limited immunity from liability for hospitals that participate in both contributing data to, as well as consulting, a National Practitioner Data Bank. The data bank contains information such as restrictions or revocations of medical staff membership and clinical privileges, malpractice payments, state licensure, and society membership actions.

Hospitals are required to submit information on reduction, suspension, denial, revocation, restriction, nonrenewal, or surrender of medical staff privileges lasting longer than 30 days. Hospitals also must report information related to malpractice payments made on behalf of licensed health practitioners. Hospitals must query the data bank every two years concerning reappointment of medical staff members and those holding clinical privileges. They also must access the bank when screening applicants for initial appointment and granting of privileges ("Data banking," 1989, p. 6). Hospitals that fail to comply with the reporting requirements of the act can face substantial penalties: fines of up to $10,000 per occurrence and loss of immunity protection for a three-year period (National Practitioner Data Bank [Title IV Regulations, Oct. 1989, pp. 5, 7]).

Although implementation of the data bank and questions about its utility and effectiveness will take several years to resolve, hospital boards should be aware of hospital responsibilities related to the bank as well as potential problems it poses. For example, some experts are concerned that the data bank will have a chilling effect on medical staff participation in the credentialing process and may even worsen rather than improve the way credentialing is conducted ("Key problems," 1990, p. 1).

Hospital medical staff committees and hospital boards must now, more than ever before, make sure that medical staff applications and requests for privileges are handled carefully and completely. Governing boards must ensure that the hospital has in place and is using a thorough, consistent, and fair credentialing process and that trained personnel participate in both contributing information to the bank and querying and using the information appropriately for reviewing medical staff candidates.

In reaching final decisions on medical staff applicants, boards should remember that the data bank is only one source of information that should be used as part of a broader investigation into the candidate's capability and competency to practice. Even though the data bank may indicate a clean record, a more extensive investigation might uncover a different picture of the candidate. To help protect themselves and their hospitals from potential liability, boards must rely on sources other than the data bank, such as internal hospital quality and risk management information. Careful review and interpretation of data bank information is required by all participants in the credentialing process to ensure that final decisions on each applicant are made first in the best interests of the patients the hospital serves, and then the practitioner.

Regulatory Mandates

In addition to legal and legislative imperatives, the Joint Commission on Accreditation of Healthcare Organizations also specifies the board's ultimate accountability for medical staff appointment and privileges delineation. As mentioned in chapter 3, the Joint Commission standards require the medical staff executive committee to make recommendations for approval by the governing body regarding mechanisms to review credentials and delineate individual clinical privileges. The standards also require board approval of medical staff recommendations regarding individual medical staff membership and specific clinical privileges for each eligible practitioner.

These legal, legislative, and regulatory mandates clearly indicate the board's accountability for medical staff appointment and privileges delineation. Yet many boards that continue to "rubber stamp" their medical staff's recommendations do so not only to avoid conflict but also because they simply do not understand how the credentialing process works and how the board can most effectively participate in it. Because they are not familiar with the process and are not aware of the information that typically is reviewed on each candidate, many trustees are uncomfortable asking questions or seeking additional information before making final decisions on medical staff recommendations.

The next section of this chapter discusses the key players and their roles in credentialing and reviews the steps in the process to help you gain a basic understanding of how to meaningfully participate in this critical quality assurance responsibility.

The Basics of Credentialing

Credentialing consists of two separate processes: appointment to the medical staff and delineation of clinical privileges. Each process has its own objective.

The *appointment process,* which is composed of initial appointment to the medical staff and periodic reappointments thereafter, is designed to evaluate the individual practitioner's *capability* to practice at the hospital. The appointment process focuses on a review of a practitioner's education, training, licensure, certification, references, and other credentials that testify that the individual is eligible to be a member of the hospital's medical staff.

When candidates apply for medical staff membership, they generally also apply for specific privileges to practice at the hospital. The *delineation of clinical privileges process* focuses on assessing the practitioner's *competence* to treat various illnesses or perform various procedures. In granting privileges to individual physicians, the board is specifying the scope of that individual's competence to practice within his or her areas of skill and expertise (Orlikoff, 1990, p. 63).

Once physicians gain initial appointment and privileges, they enter a provisional period of medical staff membership, usually lasting six months to a year, during which their performance is monitored closely. If at the end of this time the physician and the hospital have found the experience mutually satisfactory, the physician gains full membership status and is subject to periodic reappraisal and reappointment, usually conducted at least every two years (Orlikoff and Totten, 1988, p. 15). This reappraisal may result in an alteration (restriction, expansion, or revocation) of delineated clinical privileges.

Relative Roles of Participants in the Credentialing Process

Before learning the specifics of the credentialing process, it is helpful to understand who participates in it and the roles of each participant. Each member of the hospital leadership team—the governing board, the medical staff, and the hospital management group—has a role to play.

As you might suspect, the bulk of the review and analysis of a physician's capability and competency is conducted by the *medical staff* because a physician's peers are best able to assess and make recommendations regarding the practitioner's background and expertise. It is the medical staff that establishes the applicant evaluation process in its bylaws and works with candidates to obtain appropriate information for review. Once a completed application has been received, the medical staff credentialing committee (or its equivalent) reviews the information to assess the candidate's professional competence, performance, character, and fitness and then makes a recommendation regarding the candidate. Frequently this recommendation is reviewed by the medical staff executive committee, which then sends the recommendation to the governing board.

In discharging its responsibilities for credentialing, the medical staff often relies on support from the hospital's management group. *Hospital managers* have an important role to play in ensuring that adequate staff and other resources and support are available to the medical staff to gather and verify applicant information. Hospital executives also can facilitate the flow of information, such as hospital quality assurance and risk management data, that should be used in evaluating candidates. Finally, the hospital chief executive officer should help facilitate the flow of medical staff recommendations and supporting documentation to the governing board and help establish a collaborative process between the board and medical staff for reaching final decisions on medical staff candidates.

Ultimately it is up to the *governing board* to render final decisions on each medical staff applicant. Although the governing board does not actively participate in data collection and validation for each candidate, the board is responsible for ensuring that the medical staff bylaws provide for a credentialing procedure and that this procedure is in fact conducted thoroughly and consistently for each candidate. The board must ensure that appropriate information on each candidate has been received and reviewed (see the next section) and that all questions regarding the applicant have been satisfactorily answered. The board must make sure it understands the medical staff's recommendation and compares it against the criteria established in the medical staff's credentialing procedure. Finally, the board must make a determination on staff membership and privileges for each candidate (Orlikoff, 1990, pp. 63–64).

The Appointment and Privileges Delineation Processes

Trustees who understand the information received and reviewed during the appointment and privileges delineation processes are best able to participate knowledgeably and meaningfully in reaching final decisions on applicants. This section reviews initial appointment and reappointment to the medical staff and discusses the granting of medical staff privileges in more detail.

The Initial Appointment Process and Provisional Membership

The hospital often has its first opportunity to become familiar with a practitioner during the initial appointment process. Much of the information reviewed during this process is supplied from outside sources, so the medical staff and board must be especially thorough and diligent in obtaining and reviewing all relevant and appropriate information. The essential minimum information that should be received and reviewed on each candidate is:

- Validation of licensure in all states that apply
- Evidence of completed training, including undergraduate and medical school education, and residency, fellowship, or other training, if claimed
- Disciplinary actions by previous hospitals, professional societies, or specialty boards, if any
- Current good standing at other hospitals
- Current and adequate malpractice insurance
- Valid board certification, if claimed or required by the hospital
- Satisfactory recommendations regarding professional performance, clinical skills, ethical character, ability to work with others
- Statement of health history, including substance abuse or chronic illnesses, if any
- Malpractice claims history
- Privileges granted at other hospitals and evidence of special training and experience, especially in conducting high-risk or unusual procedures

The board should make sure that any questions regarding the practitioner's capabilities are answered satisfactorily prior to initial appointment. The burden of proof to obtain medical staff membership resides with the applicant and, therefore, this is the best time to catch any potential problems. It is usually much easier to prevent a physician with a questionable background from joining the medical staff than to remove a physician once he or she has become a medical staff member.

Once the initial appointment process has been successfully completed, the applicant undergoes a period of provisional membership on the medical staff. This period, though frequently underused, is the one opportunity that allows the hospital to monitor the physician in action and to gain firsthand experience with physicians *prior to* admitting them to the medical staff. Hospitals that use the provisional period well can acquire valuable information that will help the board make a more informed decision about whether to confer full membership status or grant the privileges requested by physician applicants. For these reasons, your board should ensure that the medical staff bylaws specify a monitoring process to be used during the provisional period and that information about physician performance during this period be submitted to the board prior to making final decisions about admitting physicians to the medical staff.

The Reappointment Process

Each medical staff member must reapply for medical staff membership and undergo a reappointment process at least every two years. This time, the emphasis is on actual physician performance at the hospital during the past two years. In addition to the type of information reviewed during initial appointment, the hospital should now rely on several sources of internal information in assessing candidates.

For example, mortality statistics, infection rates, or malpractice claims can be provided by the hospital's quality assurance and risk management department. The board and medical staff also have access to a variety of performance-specific information. Compliance with hospital and medical staff bylaws, rules, and regulations; patterns of adverse clinical outcomes; and reduction or revocation of privileges are examples of some of the performance indicators that should be considered during reappointment. Such data should be carefully gathered and considered because the burden of proof lies with the hospital in the event reappointment is denied. Ultimately, a thorough, fair, and consistent approach to appointment and reappointment is in the best interest of the hospital, its practitioners, and its patients.

The Privileges Delineation Process

Generally practitioners will submit a request for medical staff privileges along with their applications for appointment. The delineation of privileges is practitioner specific and defines the types of illnesses that can be treated or the procedures that can be performed. Privileges usually are developed by each clinical department in the hospital using one of several approaches. They can be specified by practitioner's specialty, patient risk category, lists or groups of procedures and diseases, or combinations of these. The specificity required for delineating privileges may vary for each hospital based on its size, complexity, and staffing.

The process for granting clinical privileges also requires review of the appointment information listed previously, with special emphasis on assessing the candidate's competency to treat the diseases or perform the procedures specified. In assessing the candidate's level of expertise, the medical staff may review the individual's initial and continuing education, overall use of privileges previously granted, volume of cases seen or procedures performed, and specific outcome indicators (unplanned returns to surgery or number of missed diagnoses). After the review is completed, the medical staff can make any of a number of recommendations, including to approve, deny, revoke, restrict, reduce, suspend, or expand the practitioner's privileges, as appropriate.

Boards that participate effectively in the appointment and privileges delineation processes balance their responsibility for ensuring quality care with the physician's interest in practicing at the hospital. If the board decides, for example, to deny, modify, or revoke a medical staff member's privileges, it must do so according to the hospital's bylaws and be consistent with constitutional or common law requirements of due process. These requirements usually call for fair and consistent application of criteria based on professional standards of care, the legitimate objectives of the hospital, and the character and ethical behavior of the applicant (Orlikoff and Totten, 1988, p. 15).

Economic Credentialing

Although most credentialing processes largely focus on the *clinical* skills of the physician, some recent court cases have upheld denial of medical staff privileges based on *economic* results of the physician's practice, such as overutilization of hospital resources. This is called *economic credentialing*, and hospitals that set resource use standards must include them in the hospital bylaws, apply them fairly and consistently to all practitioners, and give those whose practice patterns deviate from the standards an opportunity to comply.

To understand the reason for economic credentialing, consider the following situation. A physician at your hospital is up for reappointment to the medical staff and meets all the clinical and administrative criteria for reappointment; in other words, the physician's quality of care is good. However, the physician consistently *costs* the hospital huge sums of money by requesting extra tests and treatments. The physician also has a history of extended patient stays, which results in frequent payment denials by Medicare, insurers, and other third-party payers. Now imagine that your hospital is in economic trouble and has a negative operating margin.

Clearly, in this situation the hospital must act to control the physician's inappropriate resource use, which is costing the hospital money it can ill afford to lose. If counseling and education—the first-line approaches—do not change the physician's expensive behavior, then the hospital might establish criteria to conduct economic credentialing in the future.

Bear in mind, however, that the issue of economic credentialing is a controversial one that is likely to cause concern among physicians. It is an issue that can generate litigation and, if improperly approached, liability for the hospital and the board. Yet it also is an issue that many hospitals and boards likely will find they must confront in the near future (Blum, 1990, p. 30).

Common Problems in Credentialing

Now that you know the basic process of credentialing, you also should know about problems that commonly occur in credentialing. The first and foremost problem is confusion between the role of the medical staff and the role of the board. This role confusion frequently results in disagreement, conflict, and ineffective credentialing.

In a nutshell, here is the difference in roles: The medical staff does the actual work of credentialing; that is, it develops criteria, evaluates applicants, and makes recommendations. The board, on the other hand, makes certain that the medical staff has done it right and has used the same process consistently for each candidate; that is, the board reviews medical staff recommendations against credentialing criteria, verifies that the recommendations are appropriate, and makes final decisions.

The next problem is that even if relative roles are known and understood, the medical staff credentialing criteria are often so vague that it is impossible for the board to do its job meaningfully. Most medical staff criteria relate to administrative issues such as licensure, meeting attendance, and the like. A physician's clinical skill and performance, on the other hand, usually are determined by the particular medical staff department head.

In most hospitals, the critical judgment of the medical staff department head is a subjective one. If the credentialing process, and specifically the privileges delineation process, relies too heavily on the subjective judgment of medical staff department heads, then it is impossible for the board to verify the appropriateness of a particular recommendation *or* to ensure that the process is equally and consistently applied to all applicants.

How can the board know the appropriateness of a subjective judgment—in essence, what went on in the mind of a medical staff department head or credentials committee? How does the board know the department head or credentials committee would make the same recommendation for two different physician applicants if both had similar clinical skills and performance records but different social or economic relationships with these evaluators? How can the board know that certain department heads are *not* making negative credentialing recommendations when they *should* be, because they fear being sued by the physician applicant? Unfortunately the answer to these and similar questions is that, under the vast majority of credentialing systems, *the board simply cannot know.*

Often there is no evidence that the *past practice* of renewal applicants is systematically evaluated and relied on by medical staff department heads and credentials committees to recommend privileges renewal, expansion, restriction, or revocation. This also is due to the subjectivity of the process.

A similar problem is that there rarely is evidence that the results of the hospital's quality assurance activities are meaningfully integrated into the reappointment and privileges renewal process. Each physician who reapplies for membership and privileges has had two years' worth of quality assurance monitoring and evaluation and peer review of the quality of his or her care. This is *precisely* the information that the reappointment process should rely on. Unfortunately it rarely does. What is the point of the hospital conducting these activities if the information they yield is not used?

To summarize, the most common credentialing problems are lack of definition of relative roles between the medical staff and the board; vagueness of medical staff criteria relating to clinical performance of applicants, or subjectivity of the process; failure to systematically evaluate past practice of the applicant; and failure to objectively integrate results of quality assurance and peer review activities into the process. These common problems usually will undermine a hospital's medical staff credentialing system, thus rendering it ineffective. Do any of these problems exist in your hospital's credentialing system? The next section will suggest a process to help overcome these common problems.

Reaching a Final Decision

As mentioned, the board's role is to understand and evaluate the credentialing process used by the medical staff and to reach a final decision on appointment and privileges delineation for each candidate. To understand the process and recommendations made by the medical staff, the board needs to be aware of the criteria used by the medical staff to evaluate each candidate. These criteria then can be used by the board to evaluate the medical staff's decision-making process.

Decision-making criteria should be developed jointly by the medical staff and the board, incorporated into the medical staff bylaws, and consistently applied to each applicant. Using such criteria can help make the process of reaching a final decision more objective and can help establish a basis of fairness in consideration of all candidates.

When the board receives the medical staff's recommendation, it should be accompanied by the criteria used to evaluate the applicant and by a summary of the information received and verified by the medical staff, indicating which criteria were met. Then the board can use the decision criteria to evaluate the medical staff's review and recommendation process and to independently determine whether its final decision coincides with the medical staff's recommendation. If it does, the board can then approve the recommendation. However, if the board determines that the medical staff's decision is not consistent with the criteria, the board should reverse the recommendation in favor of a final decision that is in fact based on the criteria profile specific to each candidate. The board also should direct the medical staff to follow the criteria in considering all candidates. In this way the board both verifies whether the established credentialing process has been followed and also makes a final decision that is consistent with the process and the criteria that support it (Orlikoff, 1990, pp.67–68).

This is an important point to stress. The board simply compares the medical staff recommendation for a particular applicant to that applicant's criteria profile. If the medical staff recommendation is consistent with the criteria, the board votes to approve the medical staff recommendation. If the recommendation and profile are inconsistent, *the board votes a decision that is mandated by the criteria.*

Obviously, for the credentialing process to work, there must be objective, measurable criteria for the medical staff to use in evaluating applicants and for the board to use in evaluating and voting on the recommendations of the medical staff. The next section discusses a method for developing such a criteria-based credentialing system.

A Level 1 and Level 2 Criteria System

Hospital boards and medical staffs can take a variety of approaches to developing decision criteria. A simple two-level system is one approach.

Level 1 criteria would be an essential, minimum set; that is, if even one criterion is not met, the candidate would not be appointed or granted privileges to practice at the hospital. Examples of such "deal-breaker" criteria are:

- Valid medical license in all states that apply
- Verification of medical school, residency, or other required training
- Adequate and current malpractice insurance
- A completed application

For those physicians reapplying for medical staff membership, these additional level 1 criteria are usually added:

- Must have attended at least 50 percent of all medical staff meetings
- Must not have delinquent medical records for more than _____ (a specified period of time)

If your hospital is like the vast majority of hospitals, only level 1 criteria are used. That is, because every single criterion must be met for an applicant to join or remain on the medical staff, *every* criterion is a potential "deal-breaker."

The problem with the level 1 approach is its inflexibility. As a result, the medical staff resists the development and use of *criteria that measure the clinical skill and performance of a physician.* It is precisely these types of criteria that should be used in the credentialing process, but most medical staff would not like the idea of a negative credentialing decision being triggered by missing *one* clinical criterion (such as a high infection rate).

This is the reason why clinical criteria are nonexistent or vague in most hospitals' medical staff credentialing systems. This is also a fundamental reason why many trustees are uncomfortable with the credentialing process; they see objective, measurable criteria used for *administrative issues* but see no such criteria for *clinical issues.* The trustees get the sense that they must blindly trust the subjective judgment of the medical staff regarding clinical issues.

A way to correct this serious flaw in a credentialing system is to create level 2 criteria. Whereas failure to meet any single level 2 criterion would not result in denial of staff appointment or privileges, failure to meet a predefined threshold, perhaps 3 of 10, would trigger a negative credentialing decision.

This level 2 criteria system allows a great deal of flexibility and thus facilitates the use of objective *clinical* criteria. Bear in mind that the medical staff would develop both the level 2 criteria *and* the criteria threshold for a negative decision. Examples of possible level 2 criteria that are primarily clinically or quality related are shown in figure 6-1.

Under this system, a board would get a criteria profile sheet for each physician applicant. It would show whether all level 1 criteria were met;

Figure 6-1. Examples of Level 2 Medical Staff Quality-Related Credentialing Criteria

1. Nosocomial (hospital-acquired) infection rates. (Note: Infection rate criteria and other quality-related criteria are usually rated in comparison to the arithmetic mean of the medical department in question. For example, a nosocomial infection rate that is *1 standard deviation* above the mean of the infection rate for the entire Internal Medicine Department can be used as a level 2 criterion.)

2. Inpatient mortality rates.

3. Surgical wound infection rates.

4. Unplanned returns to operating room; this can be expressed as a set percentage of a surgeon's cases or can be compared to the mean of the department.

5. Maximum cesarean section rates (as a percentage of an individual's cases).

6. Perioperative mortality rates.

7. Neonatal mortality rates.

8. Rates of unplanned readmissions to hospital.

9. Rates of unplanned transfers or returns to special care units.

10. Patient complaint rates.

11. Number of malpractice claims or filed lawsuits; either as an absolute number per year or as a statistical comparison to other physicians in the same department or on the entire medical staff.

12. Adequate use of privileges previously granted; frequency criteria for procedure-specific privileges delineation.

13. Abusive or disruptive behavior. (Note: This must be more specifically defined, such as arguments with patients, arguments with staff, sexual harassment of patients or staff, assaults on either patients or staff, inebriation or intoxication, or drug use. Also, this criterion is expressed as a defined maximum number of occurrences and *not* as a comparative percentage—for example: two instances of abusive or disruptive behavior during a 12-month period.

14. Department-specific requirements for continuing medical education *in addition to* those requirements for medical staff membership.

---

what the level 2 criteria threshold was for negative action—missing 4 out of 8 or 3 out of 7 criteria, for example; which level 2 criteria were met; and the recommendation of the medical staff. The board then simply *compares* the recommendation for each candidate to that candidate's *criteria profile* and votes accordingly. If the recommendation is consistent with the criteria profile, the board votes to approve the recommendation. If inconsistent, the board votes *consistent with the criteria* and then communicates with the medical executive committee to determine why their recommendation was inconsistent with the established criteria.

A sample level 1 and level 2 evaluation form is shown in figure 6-2. This form, initially developed and used by the medical staff, shows established criteria thresholds, which level 1 and level 2 criteria were met or not met, and the recommendation of the medical staff regarding Dr.

Figure 6-2. Sample Level 1 and Level 2 Evaluation Form

Reappointment: Dr. Sam Scalpel General Surgeon	Level 1: Must meet all Level 2: Must meet 4 or more	
Level 1 Criteria	**Evaluation Meets**	**Evaluation Does Not Meet**
1. Has a valid medical license (expiration date: 1992)	X	
2. Has current and valid medical malpractice insurance ($1 million/$3 million coverage; expiration date: 1992)	X	
3. Attended a minimum of 50% of all medical staff and medical staff department meetings	X	
4. Had no medical records delinquent for more than 30 days	X	
Total	4	

Level 2 Criteria		
1. Surgical wound infection rate less than or equal to 10% of all cases	X	
2. Unplanned returns to operating room less than or equal to 1 standard deviation above the mean for all surgeons in the department		X
3. Mortality rate less than or equal to 2 standard deviations above the mean for all surgeons in the department	X	
4. Abusive/disruptive behavior (documented arguments with or assaults on patients and/or staff) occurred 4 or fewer times in the past 2 years	X	
5. Patient complaints occurred in 7% or less of all cases treated		X
6. Four or fewer malpractice suits or claims occurred in the past 2 years		X
7. Obtained at least 30 hours of category 1 continuing medical education (CME) in the past 2 years	X	
8. During the past 2 years has performed at least 1 of all procedures for which privileges are currently held	X	—
Total	5	3

Recommended for reappointment: Yes X   No ___

Richard Pritchard, M·D · Chief, Department of Surgery

Neville Melville, M.D.   Chair, Medical Staff Credentialing Committee

Sara O'Hara, M.D.   Chair, Medical Executive Committee

Scalpel's reappointment. The board can easily review this form, make sure the medical staff's evaluation and recommendation are consistent with the criteria thresholds, and then vote. As the medical staff and the board gain experience in developing and using this evaluation method, new criteria may be added or existing criteria tightened or revised.

The level 1 and level 2 criteria system, developing various levels of criteria and then assigning different decision outcomes to each level, has several advantages. Such criteria make the decision-making process more objective, consistent, and verifiable by the board; furthermore, they help ensure that several important criteria, which alone may not be actionable, nevertheless are considered during the evaluation process. The level 1 and level 2 criteria system also allows the integration of critically important clinical and quality criteria into the credentialing process. Joint development and use of the level 1 and level 2 criteria system also can lead to more informed, productive, and improved relationships throughout the hospital leadership team.

Conclusion

Hospital governing boards, executives, and medical staffs that understand and adhere to the credentialing process and their respective roles in it can most effectively ensure a medical staff that is capable and competent to provide high-quality patient care. You and members of your board must remember that your primary responsibility in the credentialing process is to ensure that a criteria-based evaluation process exists and is being applied fairly and consistently to each medical staff candidate. Once you are assured that such a process is being used in the hospital, then the board can review the medical staff's recommendation against the established criteria, verify that the recommendation is appropriate, and make a final decision for each applicant.

Although the medical staff initiates establishment of the evaluation criteria and thresholds for decision making, your board should ensure that the criteria developed address administrative as well as clinical or quality-related issues as indicated in the level 1 and level 2 system described in this chapter. Such a system is the only way you can ensure thorough, objective, consistent, and fair evaluation of each candidate. And it is this approach to the credentialing process that leads to successful fulfillment of this critical board quality assurance responsibility.

References

Blum, J. Study examines role of hospital boards in physician evaluation: economic credentialing may raise legal, political issues. *Modern Healthcare* 20(3); 30–31, Jan. 22, 1990.

Data banking. *QRC Advisor* 5(12):1, 6–8, Oct. 1989.

Joint Commission on Accreditation of Healthcare Organizations. *Report on the Joint Commission's Survey of Relationships among Governing Bodies, Management, and Medical Staffs in United States Hospitals.* Chicago: JCAHO, 1987.

Key problems of the National Practitioner Data Bank. *Staff Privileges Report* 2(12):1–2, Jan. 1990.

National Practitioner Data Bank for Adverse Information on Physicians and Other Health Care Practitioners. 45 CFR Part 60 of §§401–432 of the Health Care Quality Improvement Act of 1986. Pub. L. 99-660, 100 Stat. 3784–3794, as amended by §402 of Pub. L. 100–177 Stat. 1007-1008 (42 U.S.C. 11101-11152).

Orlikoff, J. *Quality from the Top: Working with Hospital Governing Boards to Assure Quality Care—A Guide for Quality Assurance Professionals.* Chicago: Pluribus Press, 1990.

Orlikoff, J., and Totten, M. Medical staff appointments and privileges: key role of the governing board. *Trustee* 41(4):14–15, Apr. 1988.

Patrick v. Burget, 108 S.Ct. 1658 (1988).

Chapter 7

Improving the Board's Information about Quality

Introduction

Information about quality is important to your board—not just the content and timeliness of information, but the appropriateness of it as well. Information is appropriate only when it helps the group receiving it to do its job effectively. Because different groups within the hospital perform different jobs, it is logical that the information required by each group to do its job will also be different.

To effectively oversee your hospital's quality of care and contribute to its improvement, your board needs information about quality that is appropriate to the role and function of the board. Why? Quite simply, because the information that your board receives will greatly influence how your board understands and addresses the issue of quality in your hospital.

This is a crucial point. The level of detail, the format, the content, and the frequency with which quality-related information is presented to your board will actually structure how your board responds to the information and oversees the quality of care in your hospital. If your board does not have a defined role regarding its responsibility and involvement in quality, the quality-related information your board receives or does not receive will actually structure its role in quality on a de facto basis. Although this is not an appropriate way for a board's role in quality to be determined, this is the way it happens in many hospitals throughout the country.

Clearly the appropriate approach is to first define and clarify the role of the board regarding quality. Then the board's role in quality should be defined in relation to the role of other groups within the hospital—the medical staff, management, and the board quality committee, for example. Next the information the board receives should be structured to flow from and to support the defined role of the board. Only then will the information actually facilitate the board's effectively performing its quality-related functions.

The need for appropriate information strikes at the very heart of the issue of the distinction in role and function between board, management, and medical staff. If you think about it, you will clearly see that the board, medical staff, and management have very different jobs relating to quality. Yet if each group receives the same information at about the same time and in the same manner, what is the difference between what each group does? The answer is that there will be little, if any, perceptible difference in function between the different groups.

This is one of the main contributors to the frequently heard problem of a board being overinvolved in "management," or a board that meddles in the affairs of the medical staff, or a board that is not "governing appropriately." First, in these situations there usually has been no definition of the relative roles of the three groups regarding quality (or other issues at hand). Second, there is consequently no difference in the *information* that the three groups receive. Thus it is difficult to see how the functions of the groups are, or should be, different from one another.

Think of it this way. If a board is given *management* information, it will probably start performing functions that are appropriate to management. If a board is given *clinical* information, it will be drawn to performing functions that are the domain of the medical staff. Conversely, if a board is given *no* information or *meaningless* information, it likely will do nothing at all. For boards to govern effectively, they must be provided with effective governance information. This is especially true in the area of quality.

This chapter addresses the issue of how to make certain that your board receives meaningful *governance information* regarding quality. It reviews how to use what you now know about the issue of quality to help define or refine the role your board plays in quality of care; to define and structure the types, formats, and frequency of information your board receives about quality; and to effectively respond to that information. In this way your board will be well on the road to effectively overseeing your hospital's quality of care.

Information about Quality versus Information about the QA Program

As you and your board begin to consider what information to receive about quality, it is important to address two different but closely related categories of information: information about your hospital's *quality of care* and information about its *QA Program and related activities.* At first glance you might not see much of a difference between these two categories of information. The difference is indeed subtle, but extremely important for you and your board to understand.

Much of the information your board receives regarding quality will be generated by the activities of the QA Program. Thus if the QA Program, or parts of it, are not functioning effectively, it will not generate meaningful information about your hospital's quality of care. In other words, if your QA Program and related activities are not up to speed, your board cannot trust the information about quality that is generated by them.

For example, assume that your hospital's Department of Surgery does not have an effective monitoring and evaluation process or a surgical case review function. Consequently, very few problems are identified; of those that are identified, none are deemed significant enough to warrant much attention. This information is then repeatedly reported to your board as "No significant problems or patterns of problems identified in the care of surgical patients; quality of care is excellent." Is the quality of surgical care really excellent in this situation?

The answer is that you, as well as the Department of Surgery, really do not know. The quality of care may be good, but there also may be serious problems or opportunities to improve quality that are masked by the ineffective quality assessment and assurance activities. As a consequence, any such problems are overlooked, and the opportunities to improve care are not taken advantage of. Yet because "no problems or patterns of problems" are identified in surgical care, it is easy—and incorrect—to conclude there are in fact no problems in surgical care, and further, that the quality of surgical care is excellent.

In this common type of situation, the medical staff leadership, management, and the board are lulled into a false sense of security. They are led to believe that the quality of care in a particular area, or throughout the entire hospital, is good when in fact significant problems exist but are obscured by ineffective quality measurement and improvement activities. Unfortunately in these situations the problems are frequently exposed by Joint Commission accreditation surveys or malpractice claims. Threats to accreditation status and costly malpractice claims are hardly an efficient or acceptable method of accurately assessing quality of care or of assessing effectiveness of the QA Program and related activities.

Your board must avoid leaping to conclusions about quality when there have been changes or improvements in the QA Program and related activities. For example, a hospital recently improved its quality assessment and improvement activities in one of the nursing areas. Previously this area generated no problems or patterns of problems, and everyone assumed this attested to the quality of care in that area. Now, due to new quality assurance activities, that nursing area is identifying many problems, patterns of problems, and opportunities to improve the quality of care. Does this mean that the quality of care in that nursing area is deteriorating?

Hardly so. What it really means is that activities devoted to identifying problems have improved and are beginning to function effectively. In this situation, just because more problems are being identified does not mean that quality of care is deteriorating. An accurate assessment of trends in the quality of care in this area cannot be made until more information is gathered over time by the improved quality assurance activities in that area. This information would demonstrate the correction of problems and improvements in care, as well as track trends in problems.

Thus it is easy (and quite common) for boards to mistakenly believe that the quality of care in a particular area, or in the whole hospital, is good when in fact that care has problems that have not been identified because the QA Program and related activities function ineffectively. Conversely and less frequently, other boards may be equally mistaken in believing that the quality of care is deteriorating when in fact they are simply receiving better, more reliable information from recently improved quality assessment and improvement activities.

Exercise continual vigilance to make certain that your board does not fall into either one of these common traps. To do this, learn to distinguish information about quality from information about the effectiveness of your QA Program and related activities. Further, learn to identify when these types of information overlap so as to avoid leaping to conclusions or being lulled into a false sense of security. The best way to do this is simply to ask questions about the information your board receives and make certain that your board receives information that relates to both issues. Questions you should ask about quality-related information presented to the board include:

- Does this information relate to quality of care, to effectiveness of one of more quality assurance and improvement processes, or both?
- If this information relates to quality of care, how was the information generated?
- Does the quality assurance process that generated the information function effectively (that is, can we trust the information)?

Your board is ultimately responsible for *both* the quality of care in your hospital and the effectiveness of your QA Program and related activities. If the QA Program does not function effectively, it will not generate meaningful or reliable information about quality. By separating information that relates to quality of care from information that relates to effectiveness of the QA Program and activities—and by identifying those situations when the information addresses both issues—your board will be much less likely to accept false conclusions.

Inadequate Quality Reports to the Board

The only thing worse than a board that receives no reports on its hospital's quality of care is a board that receives bad reports. Think back to the last several reports your board received regarding quality-related issues. Could you understand them? Did they give a clear, succinct, overall picture of your hospital's quality of care? Did they facilitate board action to improve the quality of care or the effectiveness of related activities? If you answered no, you are by no means alone.

A frequent complaint among hospital trustees is, "I rarely understand the quality reports my board receives, and when I do I am not sure what the board is supposed to *do* about them." Most often the problem here is not with the board but with the quality-related reports sent to the board. Because this chapter addresses how to make certain that your board receives effective quality-related reports, it is useful to review the many characteristics of bad or ineffective quality-related reports to boards, and the reasons behind them.

Lack of Governance Information

Perhaps the most common flaw in quality reports to boards is that they are not framed by an explicitly defined statement of the board's role in quality, quality assurance, and related activities. Therefore these reports cannot help the board discharge its role; that is, they do not provide governance information. This is because the concept of hospital governance has not been defined and distinguished from those of management and medical staff.

In relation to your board's oversight of the medical staff credentialing process, chapter 6 made a basic distinction between the role of the board and the role of the medical staff with regard to credentialing: The medical staff *does* the actual evaluation of the applicants; the board *makes certain the medical staff has done it right.* This simple role distinction then frames both the information that flows to the board as well as the actions the board might appropriately take in response to that information. Hence from that simple clarification in roles flows the process of communicating information to the board that allows it to compare the recommendations of the medical staff to the criteria profile of each applicant. The board discharges its role and responsibility by verifying that the medical staff has made appropriate recommendations for each applicant.

What about those situations where the role distinction between board and medical staff regarding credentialing has not been made? There is no guidance for what information should flow to the board; equally important, no guidance directs how the board should respond to the information it receives. This contributes significantly to the "rubber-stamp" nature of the board's decision regarding medical staff credentialing. This same situation, applied to the board's oversight of quality, is a main reason that boards also frequently simply "rubber stamp" the quality-related reports they receive.

A board with an explicitly defined role statement in the area of quality defines and specifies what quality-related information it needs to do its job. In this way, the board is *directing* the information it will receive. Conversely, a board with no defined role statement is usually *directed by* the information it receives. Thus it is difficult for such boards to effectively oversee their hospital's quality and QA Program because they are not actually directing quality-related activities but are being directed by them.

Absence of Meaningful Data Analysis

Another common flaw with quality-related reports to boards is that they provide a lot of data but little useful information. Again this relates to the difference between governance information and management and clinical information. Quality-related data presented in many board reports might be very useful to a medical staff committee or the quality assurance committee, but they often have little meaning to the board. Here the word *data* means raw numbers or simple statistics. *Information,* however, is clear analysis that shows what the data mean.

For example, boards are often provided data with no point of comparison. This is often referred to as *numerator* data without *denominator* data. Consider the following hypothetical statement from a board report: "The hospitalwide mortality rate for the month of June was 5 percent." What does this mean? Is it high or low, good or bad? How should the board respond?

Now consider this statement: "The 1990 hospitalwide mortality rate for June was 5 percent; for May, 5.5 percent; for April, 5.7 percent; for the first quarter of 1990, 6 percent; for all of 1989, 7 percent." This hypothetical statement provides the board with information that is more meaningful because it has a point of clear comparison. In this example, the board is better able to make an intelligent judgment about this particular aspect of the quality of care and determine if it needs to request further information or to take other action.

Another reason that the second statement above is a better example of effective governance information is that it also provides the board with longitudinal information, whereas the first provided only cross-sectional information. *Longitudinal information* is that collected over a long period of time. It allows a board to see trends, to consider problems in perspective, and to get a better overall picture of the quality of care and the effectiveness of quality assurance and related activities.

Cross-sectional information, on the other hand, tends to be disjointed and less clear because it is taken from a limited period of time (for example, the mortality rate in June). Consequently, cross-sectional information can often mask subtle trends in problems. For example, consider a medical department that has an unusual quality problem that on several occasions has almost caused serious injury to patients but has never had more than one such occurrence every other month. If this medical department's quality is examined by the medical staff on a monthly basis—and *only* on a monthly basis—it is unlikely that the problem will be spotted. The medical staff or the board, reviewing only the information from one month (cross-sectional information), might miss the problem altogether or rationalize its occasional occurrence as infrequent (based on one month's data) and acceptable. On the other hand, by examining the same information from the past year, the problem will become evident and will elicit corrective action.

Inappropriate Reporting

Perhaps one of the most common problems in providing quality-related reports to boards involves sending a board sets of meeting minutes. Minutes of last month's meetings of the medical executive committee, the hospitalwide QA committee, and the board QA committee, for example, are often sent to the board *as the actual quality report.* This is perhaps the biggest waste of time imaginable for a board.

Think back to your board materials and answer this question honestly. If your packet includes minutes from meetings of committees you do not belong to, do you read them? If you answer yes (if so, you are in a distinct minority), do those minutes provide your board with meaningful governance information regarding quality and quality assurance? Do they facilitate effective board action to improve quality? Do they even facilitate board oversight of the effectiveness of the function of the particular committee or group? In the vast majority of situation, the answer is no.

For these and other reasons it is wholly inappropriate for your board to receive meeting minutes as the primary vehicle for quality-related reports. Minutes may, however, be provided to your board as background to support quality-related reports. But even in this situation, minutes are of limited value in reporting quality-related information to your board or in eliciting effective and appropriate responses from your board.

Information Overload

As indicated by the preceding examples, most ineffective quality reports do not provide sufficient information to the board. This tends to elicit complacency, lack of oversight and critical questioning, and "rubber stamping" by the board. The flip side, however, is the quality-related report that is ineffective because it contains *too much information*.

In this less common but equally damaging situation, the unfortunate board receiving these reports finds itself buried in information about quality and quality assurance. Most boards respond to this in one of two equally inappropriate ways. Some boards, dazed at the voluminous and often incomprehensible quality-related reports, simply take them as evidence that their hospital really is providing good-quality care. "After all," trustees on these boards may think, "look how much paper, how many studies, how many numbers, are being generated; it must mean that our quality of care is fine and our QA Program effective." The common result of quality-related reports that inflict information overload on the trustees who receive them is that the board simply "tunes out" both the reports and the issue of quality.

There is another response to quality-related information overload that is less common, but that usually causes many problems. This is the situation where the board responds to excessive information by becoming inappropriately overinvolved in quality, quality assurance, and related activities. Can a board be overinvolved in quality? Certainly, when its involvement transcends the boundaries of governance and enters the domains of management or clinical medicine without good reason (for example, when management or the medical staff abdicates its responsibility and fails to discharge its role in quality, thus forcing the board to step in to address the situation). Please understand that your board cannot be *overcommitted* to quality, but it can be inappropriately *overinvolved* in quality, quality assurance, and related functions.

In these situations, the board that receives too much information is usually receiving management or clinical information. The board is then tempted to perform management or clinical functions—in which case it can easily cause tension and conflict among itself, management, and the medical staff over the issue of quality. This, of course, is counterproductive to quality-improvement efforts, because they require sincere top-level commitment and effective teamwork.

Other Common Problems

Other common flaws in quality reports to boards include:

- Reports that only provide information on the process of the QA Program and related activities, but not on the outcomes of care

- Reports that routinely present insignificant quality-related issues but hide or gloss over significant quality problems or issues
- Reports that contain meaningful information but are presented in formats that are unclear, disorganized, or actually prevent the board from understanding the information (long narrative reports, extensive tables in small print, extensive use of esoteric clinical language that has not been defined for the board)

All of the common problems with quality-related reports to boards discussed in this section actually serve to *hinder* a board from effectively overseeing and improving the quality of care and the effectiveness of the quality assurance and quality improvement activities. The more problems present in the quality-related reports to the board, the more problems there will be in the board's involvement in, and oversight of, quality and quality assurance.

Many common problems in quality-related reports to boards were discussed in this section. How many of these problems do you recognize in the quality-related reports your board receives?

Defining the Role of the Board

There are many reasons for your board to have a clearly defined, written statement of its role in quality of care and related activities. These include clarifying the role of the board for new members of the board (as well as reminding experienced members); clarifying the role of the board for members of the medical staff and management; developing a clear distinction between the role and responsibility of the board in quality of care and the role and responsibility of the medical staff and management; and providing a framework for the information that will be communicated to the board about quality and quality assurance, as well as for how the board will respond to that information.

Because boards differ and govern hospitals with different characteristics, each board will probably have a unique quality role statement. Your board must develop and approve a quality role statement that is tailored to your board and hospital.

To be effective, a statement of a board's role in quality of care should cover several points:

- The commitment of the hospital to quality care
- The responsibility of the board for quality and for maintaining and ensuring the hospital's commitment to quality
- The responsibility of the board to oversee the activities of the medical staff

- The responsibility of the board to oversee the hospital's QA Program and quality improvement activities
- How the board will be informed of and involved in quality, quality assurance, and medical staff affairs
- How the board can act to maintain and improve quality, and to maintain and improve effective quality assurance and quality improvement activities.

Again, each board's quality role statement will be different and may emphasize different points. For example, if your hospital has or is about to embark on a massive continuous quality improvement or total quality management effort (discussed in chapter 9), the board's role in that effort should be spelled out in the quality role statement. If the board has a standing committee that addresses quality and related issues, then the board's quality role statement should state this and spell out the relative role and responsibility of the committee in relation to the board.

The following sample statement (Orlikoff, 1990, pp. 123–24) describes a board's role in quality:

The XXX hospital is committed to providing quality care to all of its patients, and it is the governing board's responsibility to ensure that the hospital fulfills that commitment. The board has the ultimate responsibility for the quality of care provided by the hospital; for the hospital's quality assurance and risk management programs and all quality improvement activities; and, for oversight of the hospital's medical staff, which is primarily discharged through its oversight of, and final decisions regarding the appointments and privileges delineation of medical staff members.

The board will oversee and direct the hospital's quality assurance program and related functions by regularly monitoring specified information regarding the effectiveness of the QA Program and related functions. This information will place specific emphasis on the QA Program's effectiveness in the identification and resolution of problems in care, in the improvement in the quality of care, and in the effectiveness of the participation of the medical staff in quality assurance activities. The board will monitor to ensure that the results of clinical quality assurance reviews are well and objectively integrated into the medical staff credentialing process. The board will monitor the hospital's quality of care primarily through its regular review of a number of defined quality indicators, as well as other appropriate information.

Overall, it is the role of the board to monitor the quality assurance and credentialing processes of the hospital to ensure that they function effectively. The board will take action when it determines these processes to be ineffective and therefore in need of improvement. Similarly, it is the role of the board to monitor the quality of care and to take action when there are negative trends in that care or when the quality of care is in need of improvement.

You may think that role statement a bit wordy and vague to be meaningful for your board, or you may think it appropriate and useful. Whatever your sense of the sample role statement, it is important that the role of your board in quality and quality assurance be clear so that it can be written down and understood by all members of your board, as well as medical staff and management. The statement then serves as a reference point for all of the board's activities and efforts in quality of care and its improvement.

Once constructed, the quality role statement should be incorporated into the QA Plan, the board policies and procedures document, and new trustee orientation manuals. Further, your specific role statement should be routinely distributed to fellow board members to serve as a constant reminder of board responsibility, of what information the board needs to exercise that responsibility, and whether the board is in fact fulfilling its role in quality assurance.

The board's role statement can thus serve as the basis for a focused board self-evaluation with regard to quality of patient care. The ongoing process of improving the board's oversight of quality, quality assurance, and medical staff activities will then be reflected in periodic modifications and refinements in the board's role statement.

Determining Quality Indicators for the Board

Having defined the role of the board in quality and quality assurance, your board can now select a group of quality indicators that will be regularly reported to the board. The concept of the quality indicators should be mentioned in the board's quality role statement and thus should flow from the role of the board. In this way the quality indicators will be appropriate as governance information as well as reinforcement of the board's role in quality of care.

Selecting a series of quality indicators serves several purposes for the board. It develops a set format of governance information about quality that the board will routinely monitor. These indicators, taken as a whole, will provide the board with an ongoing, trend-sensitive, overall picture of its hospital's quality of care. The group of indicators will also serve to make quality more meaningful and understandable to the board. Most important, the quality indicators will facilitate effective board oversight of quality and will signal when board action is appropriate. Quality indicators for your board will help you understand what the level of quality is in your hospital and whether it is getting better or worse over time.

In order to select a number of relevant quality indicators, it is necessary to revisit the issue of your hospital's definition of quality. Chapter 4 outlined the approach to defining quality by identifying the various perspectives of quality that are valued by the hospital and its board. For each of the perspectives chosen, a number of specific indicators should be developed that address quality from that particular perspective. It is appropriate that many of the quality indicators should address medical/ clinical issues, but the indicators should address other perspectives as well. Make certain that the quality indicators for your board also reflect an emphasis on internal perspectives of quality, as opposed to focusing on external perspectives of quality.

Figure 7-1 presents a selection of potential quality indicators for the board that are separated into internal and external categories and listed by various perspectives of quality. Your board can consider this list and identify particular indicators regarded as valuable for your board to regularly review. Note that many other indicators can be developed that are not included in figure 7-1. While selecting a series of quality indicators for your board, seek input from the medical staff leadership, executive management, and the quality assurance professional. They or members of your board may suggest other valid indicators as well.

No fewer than 12 and no more than 20 indicators should be chosen for routine reporting to the board. Then as your board reviews the indicators over time, the list of specific indicators can be modified and refined. Indicators of quality that were meaningful in the past may no longer be useful if they demonstrate stable and desirable trend lines for long periods of time. These may be replaced with other quality indicators that address other aspects of quality that should receive attention.

In this way your board may develop a core group of, say, 6 to 10 indicators that are always reported to the board, and a flexible group of indicators that are presented to the board on a rotating or as-needed basis. Thus your board will constantly be scanning various indicators of your hospital's quality and will be aware of trends or developments that require attention. Over time, a universe of many board indicators may be developed, but only between 12 and 20 should be presented to your board at any one time. Your board may receive the quality indicators every meeting, every other meeting, or four times per year. To facilitate effective board oversight of quality, however, the quality indicators should not be presented to your board less frequently than once a quarter.

Please bear in mind that the quality indicators will not be the only quality-related information that is presented to your board. Your board must see to it that it also receives information that addresses the function of the QA Program and related activities, medical staff credentialing

Figure 7-1. Possible Indicators of Quality for the Board, by Internal and External Category and by Perspective of Quality

Internal Information

Medical/Clinical Perspective

- Mortality rates (hospitalwide, by department or area; examples: overall hospitalwide mortality rate, neonatal and maternal mortality rate, surgical mortality rate)
- Nosocomial infection rates (hospitalwide, by department or area; examples: overall hospitalwide nosocomial infection rate, postoperative infection rate)
- Adverse drug reactions or interactions
- Unplanned returns to surgery
- Unplanned transfers to surgery, isolation, intensive care units, or cardiac care units
- Unplanned transfers to other acute care facilities
- Hospital-incurred traumas
- Discharges against medical advice (AMAs or "elopements")
- Returns to the emergency room within 72 hours of being treated in the ER
- Readmissions to the hospital within one month of discharge
- Unplanned admissions to hospital following outpatient procedures
- Cesarean section rates
- Medication error rates (hospitalwide compared to departments or areas with higher-than-average or expected rates)

Patient/Consumer Perspective

- Patient complaints (trends by department or area, hospitalwide; pattern analyses of trends)
- Patient satisfaction survey report trends
- Average patient waiting times by department or area
- Pattern analysis of letters from patients/family members to/about hospital
- Indicators suggested by patient representative
- Trends of assaults or altercations involving patients

Staff/Employee Perspective

- Staff turnover and/or absenteeism presented by department or area
- Staff complaints (trends by department or area, hospitalwide; pattern analysis of trends)
- Staff satisfaction survey report trends
- Summaries of suggestions relating to improving quality of care, working conditions, communication, organization
- Exit interview summaries

Medical Staff Perspective

- Medical staff complaints
- Medical staff satisfaction survey report trends
- Medical staff "perception index" of quality of care (based on ratings by medical staff to standardized rating scale)

Management Perspective

- Management complaints
- Management turnover
- Management "perception index" of quality of care (based on ratings by management to standardized rating scale)

Financial (Utilization Management) Perspective

- Average length of stay (ALOS) rates (hospitalwide, by department or area; or by payer mix. Examples: hospitalwide ALOS, surgical ALOS, Medicare ALOS, Medicaid ALOS, private insured ALOS, and so forth)
- Utilization rates by physician for high-cost, low-margin procedures or diseases

Continued on next page

Figure 7-1. Continued

QA Program Process Information
- Surveys of completeness and effectiveness of monitoring and evaluation process by department
- Relative rankings of departments (medical, nursing, and ancillary) by effectiveness of problem-focused process
- Trends of corrective action and action to improve the quality of care
- Trends of relative QA Program reliance on retrospective review in relation to concurrent review
- Trends of relative QA Program focus on outcomes of care in relation to structure and process of care
- Degree of integration of results of quality assessment activities into medical staff reappointment process

Risk Management Program Information
- Pattern analyses, trends of incident reports or occurrence screens
- Summaries of malpractice claims filed
- Trends of relative focus of risk management program on iatrogenic injuries versus custodial injuries

External Information
Joint Commission on Accreditation of Healthcare Organizations Perspective
- Accreditation survey report summary (once every three years)
- Summary of Type I recommendations following survey. (These, formerly referred to as "contingencies," are the areas where the hospital has significantly failed to meet the Joint Commission standards. Serious or numerous Type I recommendations can result in a Focused Survey, where the Joint Commission returns to the hospital several months after the survey report to assess whether the hospital has improved the deficient areas; and/or, they can threaten a hospital's accreditation status)
- Focused Survey report summaries
- Joint Commission–developed quality indicators

Federal Government Perspective (Medicare)
- Annual Medicare Mortality Rate
- Denials of payments

Peer Review Organization Perspective
- PRO variance reports
- Sanctions imposed by PRO

State Perspective
- Results of State Department of Health, Hospital Licensure, or equivalent surveys
- Comparative information released by State Hospital Cost Containment and Quality Improvement Council, or equivalent, if any.

Community Perspective
- Content analysis summaries (that is, positive, negative, or neutral ratings) of newspaper and electronic media stories about or relating to the hospital
- Reports of community perception studies or polls

Hospital Insurers
- Reports of insurer loss control surveys, or risk management program assessments
- Liability insurance premium adjustments based on degree of effectiveness of risk management program or past claims history

information, and other quality-related information, such as the results of special studies or reports on the resolution of serious problems. The quality indicators for your board will be the governance information about quality that your board routinely monitors.

Establishing Thresholds for Quality Indicators

Once your board has developed an initial series of quality indicators, the next task is to select a threshold level for each indicator (most indicators will lend themselves to threshold levels, but some will not). A *threshold* is a target level or goal for each indicator that serves as a reference point for your board as it reviews the trends of each individual indicator.

For example, one of the quality indicators for your board may be the hospitalwide mortality rate. If the threshold level for the mortality rate was set at 3.5 percent of all discharges, whenever hospitalwide mortalities reach or exceed 3.5 percent of discharges, your board may facilitate action to address the issue. Thus the threshold level for each quality indicator serves as a signal to the board that the quality indicator is at (or approaching) unacceptable levels.

A good way of looking at indicator thresholds is as triggers for board action. If a particular quality indicator crosses a threshold, it should trigger action by your board. Appropriate board action will depend on the indicator and individual circumstances but may include such actions as requesting more detailed information or explanations, directing corrective action, directing additional resources to the area in question, directing changes in policies and procedures, and many others. Thresholds will make the quality indicators more meaningful to your board by quickly revealing the acceptability of the level of quality of care for each indicator, and by triggering board action when necessary.

When used appropriately, threshold levels can greatly improve the value of the quality indicators to the board as governance tools for continuously improving the quality of care. This can be achieved by modifying the threshold levels to reflect improvements in quality, or to reflect higher goals for each quality indicator. Thus you and your board should not consider the threshold levels to be static. Instead, they should be regarded as fluid and changeable, but only to set higher goals and reflect improvements in care.

Consider the example of the hospitalwide mortality rate again. If for the past six to nine months hospitalwide mortalities have been far below the 3.5 percent threshold and have been averaging 2.4 percent, it is tempting to just accept the information and congratulate yourselves for having a mortality rate that is well below your threshold. Your board can believe that your hospital has high-quality care relative to the perspective of low mortalities and do nothing, or it can try to improve this perspective of quality even more. In this case, it is appropriate for the board to tighten or lower the threshold, perhaps to 2.6 percent or so. By doing this, the board recognizes the positive trend, establishes a tighter goal to increase the sensitivity of the indicator, and also increases the focus of organizational attention to this issue, which may help mortality rates remain low and possibly facilitate further reductions in average hospital-wide mortality rates. By tightening the threshold level the board also sends the hospital a very real message of commitment to quality, which will help maintain or increase the cultural climate for quality in the organization.

Of course, like any tool, the threshold levels for quality indicators can be misused and abused. Threshold levels should never be changed to accommodate poor levels of quality or to justify negative trends in the quality of care. Look again at the example of the mortality quality indicator. The threshold is again 3.5 percent, but for the past two quarters the mortality rate has steadily risen from 3.3 percent to 4.5 percent, crossing the established threshold and staying above it. One tempting (and misguided) way of addressing this would be to change the threshold level to 4.5 percent, thus masking or justifying a negative trend in mortalities. Clearly this approach is unacceptable and counterproductive to a true quality improvement effort. Make certain that your board never allows such abuses to occur. The only time a threshold level can be acceptably relaxed is when the initial threshold level was unrealistic.

Threshold levels for quality indicators can be established in a number of ways. They can be adapted from published national, regional, or local averages when available for particular indicators. These are available from your QA professional, infection control coordinator, and so on. They can be taken from clinical averages or acceptable levels that are published by professional organizations. Internally, the average of the specific quality indicator in your hospital for the past year or so can be established as an initial threshold. Alternatively, a statistical deviation from the average can be chosen, such as 1 standard deviation from the average. Another internal method is to pick a goal for quality improvement (*Quality Letter for Healthcare Leaders*, 1989), and establish that as the indicator threshold. For example, a goal might be to reduce the patient complaint rate to 5 percent, or the Cesarean section rate to 20 percent, or the nosocomial infection rate to 3.5 percent, and so on.

All of the methods in the preceding paragraph are acceptable and appropriate for establishing initial thresholds for your board's quality indicators. It is important, however, that over time the thresholds be modified to reflect more of an internal focus than an external one. In this way your board can help ensure that your hospital adopts and maintains an internal focus and motivation for quality.

Quality Report Formats

Once your board has selected a series of quality indicators and established thresholds for them, it is time to address the issue of how those indicators and thresholds, as well as other quality-related information, will be reported to your board. Perhaps the best way of ensuring that your board is provided this important information in as meaningful and understandable a fashion as possible is to require the use of graphic formats.

Receiving the quality indicators and threshold levels in the form of graphs not only will facilitate your board's understanding of the trends in the indicators but it will also enable your board to develop a clear overall picture of your hospital's quality of care. Using graphs minimizes the use of narrative and will be clearly understandable to all the members of your board.

Figure 7-2 shows a graph of hospitalwide nosocomial infections over a period of two years. Trends are immediately discernible; it takes little time to review and understand the information contained in the graph. Even so, the governance information presented in this graph can be improved. Figure 7-3 shows that same information, this time with the addition of a threshold line.

The threshold line improves the information on the graph by clearly establishing a visual reference point for your board to use in considering the trend line. Just a glance at the graph will tell whether the threshold line has been crossed by the most recent addition of information about the indicator. If it has, your board knows that further consideration of this particular quality indicator is necessary. Questions should be asked, and perhaps action should be taken.

Figure 7-4 shows a graph of hospitalwide mortalities, but with a threshold line that is set too high (or too loose). Therefore the information presented is corrupted by an improper threshold line. It may be tempting to make all the graphs of board quality indicators demonstrate "high levels of quality" by having artificially loose thresholds, but this practice will probably deceive no one. More important, this approach will create an environment that tolerates—and subsequently elicits—poor quality. Clearly the threshold line in figure 7-4 is inappropriate and should be changed. Figure 7-5 shows that same graph with a more appropriate threshold line.

Graphic formats are also an excellent vehicle for providing the board with quality-related information other than quality indicators. For example, figure 7-6 presents a pie chart that demonstrates what areas in the hospital have generated incident reports in the past two years. What does the information tell you about this hospital's incident reporting system? Does it focus on reporting custodial or iatrogenic events? The answer

Figure 7-2. Sample Board Quality Indicator Report: Graph of Hospitalwide Nosocomial Infections

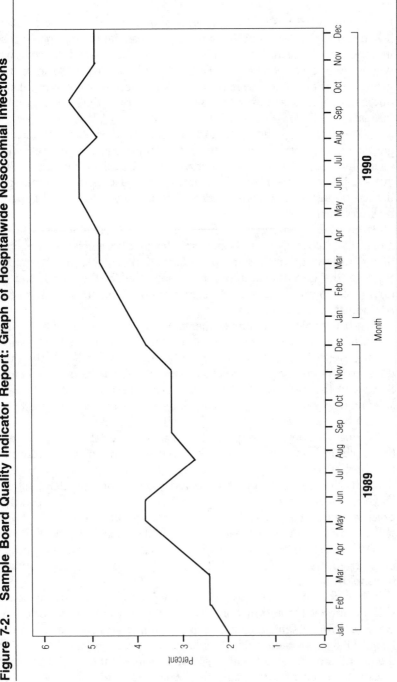

Figure 7-3. Sample Board Quality Indicator Report: Graph of Hospitalwide Nosocomial Infections, with Addition of Threshold Line

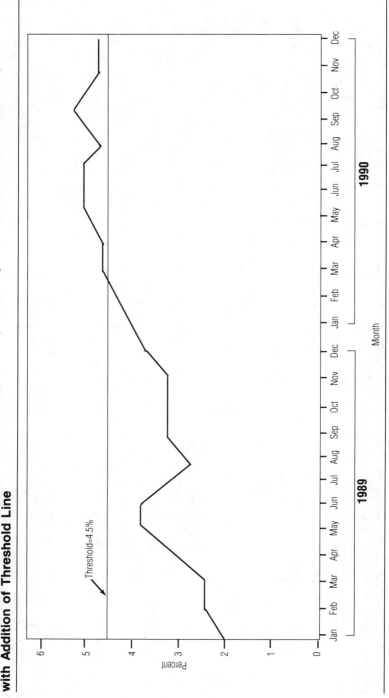

Figure 7-4. Sample Board Quality Indicator Report: Graph of Hospitalwide Mortalities as a Percentage of Discharges, with an Inappropriate Threshold Line

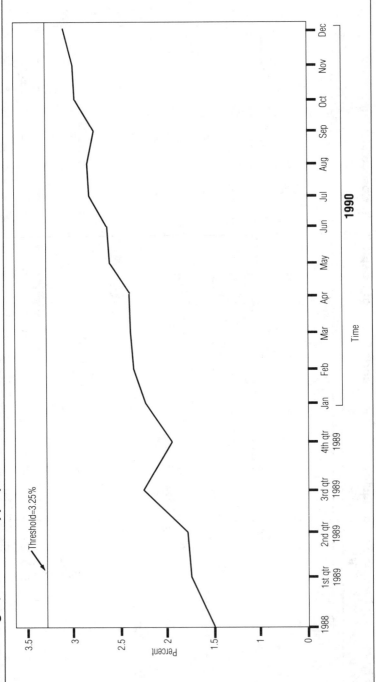

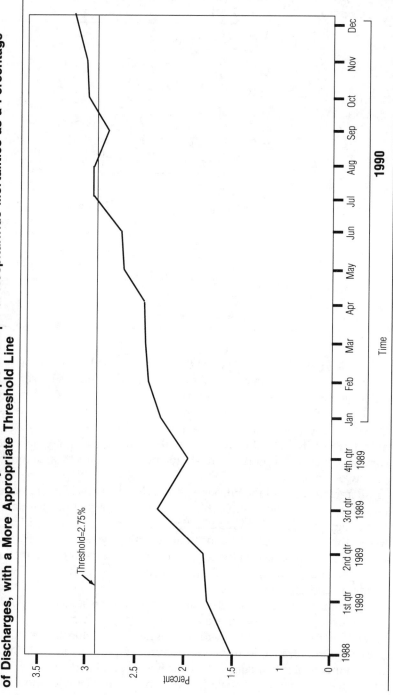

Figure 7-5. Sample Board Quality Indicator Report: Graph of Hospitalwide Mortalities as a Percentage of Discharges, with a More Appropriate Threshold Line

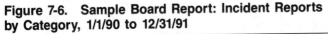

Figure 7-6. Sample Board Report: Incident Reports by Category, 1/1/90 to 12/31/91

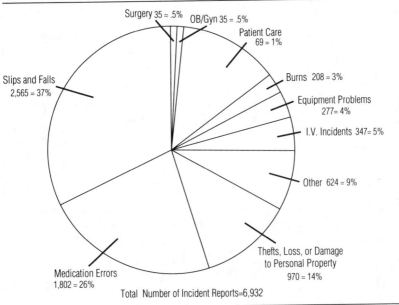

is that the graph demonstrates that the hospital's incident reporting system focuses primarily on custodial events and largely misses those medical areas that represent the highest risks to patients of iatrogenic injury.

Figure 7-6 is an example of information that helps the board to assess the effectiveness of quality-related activities, as opposed to assessing an aspect of quality itself. Figure 7-7 does this also, showing a graph that compares incident reports by area to malpractice claims by area for the past two years.

Remember, one of the purposes of your hospital's incident (or occurrence) reporting system is to detect the potential for malpractice claims *before* they are filed. The graph in figure 7-7 allows a board quickly to assess the effectiveness of the incident reporting system in its hospital. If this were a graph presented to your board, representing information from your hospital, what would it say about the effectiveness of your incident reporting system?

Graphic formats are excellent vehicles for the presentation of quality indicators, quality assurance process measures, and other quality-related information to your board. Of course, other information will be presented in narrative formats and by verbal reports. This other information that relates to quality but that is not reflected in the quality indicators (medical staff credentialing information is an example) should be

Figure 7-7. Sample Board Report: Incident Reports Compared to Malpractice Claims, 1/1/90 to 12/31/91

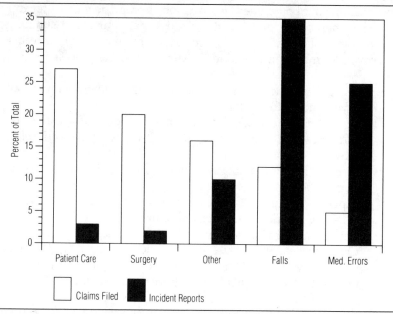

identified by your board and should become predefined parts of the routine quality reports in your board agenda materials. The use of regular report formats that facilitate the comparison of information and the tracking of trends should be encouraged. As this other quality-related information is defined and sent to your board, review it with an eye toward identifying and minimizing the typical weaknesses in quality reports discussed earlier in this chapter. Where possible, however, an emphasis on the use of graphic formats will overcome the vast majority of typical weaknesses in quality-related reports to boards.

Quality indicators with thresholds that are presented in graphic formats are excellent examples of effective governance information in the area of quality. The routine use of graphic formats for the presentation of the quality indicators and other quality-related information will dramatically increase your board's knowledge and oversight of the quality of care that your hospital provides, as well as help increase and maintain your board's commitment to quality and its improvement.

Conclusion

To effectively govern for quality, your board must receive effective governance information regarding quality. This does not happen by chance or circumstance but results from careful thought and planning regarding exactly what your board's job is in terms of quality of care and what information your board needs to do its job appropriately and effectively.

This chapter has outlined the process that your board should go through to make certain that it receives, and will continue to receive, effective governance information. To summarize, the process involves:

- Recognizing the distinction between management, clinical, and governance information
- Separating information about quality from information that addresses the effectiveness of quality assurance and related activities
- Identifying and avoiding weaknesses in past quality reports sent to your board
- Explicitly defining the role of your board in quality assurance
- Selecting a series of quality indicators
- Determining thresholds for each of the indicators
- Choosing clear and concise graphic report formats for quality information to your board and defining the other quality-related information that will regularly be reported to your board

An important addition to this process is the periodic evaluation of the process itself. Over time the board's quality role statement, the quality indicators, and other quality-related components may require revision. The key to evaluating and improving the governance information on quality is to ask how effectively it facilitates your board's performance of its job and how could it be improved.

Effective governance requires effective information. This is especially true in the area of the board's oversight of the quality of care provided by its hospital.

References

Orlikoff, J. E. *Quality from the Top: Working with Hospital Governing Boards to Assure Quality Care—A Guide for Quality Assurance Professionals.* Chicago: Pluribus Press, 1990.

Board quality indicator report. *The Quality Letter for Healthcare Leaders* 1(2):13, Sept. 2, 1989.

Chapter 8

Quality and Board Organizational Structure

Introduction

By now you may feel more comfortable about quality in general, but you also may have additional questions about how to go about achieving and maintaining effective board oversight of quality in your hospital. If you are like most trustees, many of these questions will address the issue of what organizational structures are most conducive to effective board oversight of quality and quality assurance.

Questions frequently asked by trustees include: Should the board have a quality committee (or equivalent)? If so, who should be on it? What should the committee do? Do we need a committee, or can the entire board deal effectively with the issue of quality?

If you're a trustee of a hospital that is required to have open board meetings, you might wonder how the board can consider the often sensitive issue of quality when members of the press and public are in the boardroom. This chapter will address these and other issues of organizational structure that can have significant impact on the effectiveness of your board's oversight of quality.

Defining Board Functions

Before addressing specific issues of organizational structure, it is useful to consider the broader issue of structure in relation to function. The purpose of organizational structure (board organization, board committees, committee composition, reporting relationships, committee charges, and so on) is to effectively support the function of the organization. In other words, structure should support function.

Although may seem quite logical to you, many people seem to believe that structure creates or drives function. This thinking is evidenced by those who respond to a new issue or responsibility by saying "Let's establish a committee." Just establishing a committee does not guarantee that an issue will be satisfactorily addressed. Simply creating a new structure, such as a board committee, does not in itself create or effectively support a function, such as effective board oversight of quality.

In fact, you may have noticed that committees can actually inhibit an organization from functioning effectively. Clearly you are not interested in creating or modifying board committees and other structures in your hospital that will inhibit or complicate your board's effective oversight of quality patient care. You are interested in facilitating and improving the effectiveness of your board to perform this function.

The question is how to go about making improvements effectively and efficiently. As you can guess, the answer is not simply to say "Let's establish a board quality committee." Instead, the best way is to ask several important questions. First, what is the exact function that your board performs or intends to perform regarding quality and related issues? Once that function is defined, your board can then ask the next logical question: What structure, or structures, will best facilitate your board effectively performing that function?

Thus before establishing new structures or modifying existing ones to improve their function regarding quality, the board must first have a clear sense of exactly what that function is. Unfortunately, in many hospitals structures are created first, and the function is defined later—usually by default. Consequently, many hospitals are burdened by structures that inhibit or blunt the effectiveness and efficiency of board involvement in and oversight of quality-related activities.

To avoid such poor board structures, make certain that your board has a clearly defined function regarding quality of care. (Another word for the noun *function* is *role;* the importance of the board's role statement in quality was addressed in chapter 7.) Once your board has defined its role/function, it can address the issue of how best to establish structures to perform that function and discharge that role.

Some Structural Options for Board Oversight of Quality

A board quality committee is by no means the only structural option your board can use to address quality. Although such a committee may be appropriate for many hospitals, there are many ways your board can structure (or restructure) itself to discharge its role/function. Some of these options (Orlikoff, 1990, p. 150) include the following:

- The governance role/function is performed by the entire board.
- The governance role/function is divided between the board and a quality committee (or equivalent) of the board.
- The governance role is divided between the board and one or several standing committees of the board (such as the joint conference committee).
- The governance role/function is performed by the entire board, but trustees are assigned as members (with or without vote depending on the committee and other circumstances) of standing hospital or medical staff committees dealing with quality-related issues, such as the hospitalwide QA committee, the credentials committee, the medical staff QA committee, and the medical executive committee.
- Any conceivable combination of the above options may be devised.

Before these options are discussed further in this chapter, keep in mind this important point regarding structural options: The board may divide and assign some of its functions to a board committee or other structural vehicle, but the board *can never delegate its responsibility for quality to another group or committee.*

For example, your board can delegate some of its role/function in medical staff credentialing to a committee or another group; but it cannot delegate making final decisions on the medical staff's recommendations for admission, readmission, or delineation of privileges. Similarly, the board as a whole is responsible for the quality of care in its hospital, a responsibility that cannot be delegated.

Thus the purpose of structural options is *not* to delegate this ultimate authority and responsibility of your board to another group or groups. Instead, the purpose of structural changes is to help your board do its job better, with a maximum degree of efficiency. This may involve delegating to other groups some of the support and legwork functions necessary for effective quality-related governance so that your board gets better governance information to do its job.

Rationale for a Board Quality Committee

Although the board's quality committee (QC) is called by many names (professional affairs committee, board quality improvement committee, quality oversight committee, and so forth), there are two basic questions to consider in relation to creating or refining a quality committee. The first is why will a QC help the board do its job in quality-related activities, and the second is how the QC will actually provide that help to the board. The first question involves defining the role of the QC in relation to the board; the second question involves explicitly defining exactly what the committee will do.

Consider the issue of the role of the board in quality, quality assurance, and medical staff credentialing. If your board does not have an explicitly defined role in quality, or at least a common understanding of what its job is to be, how will a committee help your board discharge that role? The answer, of course, is that a QC in this situation probably will not help at all.

So the first thing to consider is what the role of your board is with regard to quality. If your board does not have a defined role, there is no point in considering a QC or other structural alternative until you develop and adopt such a role. If your board does have a quality role statement (as was quoted in the chapter 7), then your board can logically proceed to establish the purpose, role, and function of the QC in relation to that of the board.

You may find your board is to be typical in that it has a QC but no defined role for itself in quality assurance. In this cart-before-the-horse situation, the best thing to do is to start from scratch and develop a role statement for the board, and then use that as the basis for refining the role of your QC and, if necessary, restructuring your QC. Avoid the temptation to simply formalize the implied role of the board that is framed by its relationship to the QC and how it functions, as this will likely result in a perpetuation of ineffective board oversight of quality.

Rationales for a board QC include:

- A large hospital that generates a voluminous amount of quality-related information and that needs a group to perform a legwork and information screening and refinement function
- A board that is required to have open meetings and that needs a confidential governance forum for the consideration of sensitive quality-related issues
- A board that desires to create a forum to involve members of the medical staff and management in the governance oversight of quality
- A board that is already driven by a strong committee system

One of the most common reasons for having a board QC is the voluminous amount of quality-related information that is generated by the hospital and its medical staff. Here, the board can easily find itself buried in information, spending its valuable time trying to distinguish which information is meaningful and which is meaningless. In this situation the rationale is for the QC to act as a legwork and information screening committee. The purpose of the QC is to screen the quality-related information generated by the hospital, and to send only that information that merits the attention of the full board, along with recommendations of the QC for board action.

Of course, the issue here is determining exactly what information merits the attention of the full board. This cannot be left vague or undefined, and relates to explicitly defining the role of the QC.

The Role of a Board Quality Committee

To focus the efforts of the QC and to help ensure that it effectively supports the board's role in quality of care, the role of the QC must be clearly spelled out. This description should include what information will flow to the QC and how the QC will determine what information and recommendations it sends to the full board. Next the committee should be given an annual work plan, which addresses and expresses the specific goals and objectives of the board regarding quality for the coming year.

Figure 8-1 shows a sample description of the role/function of a quality committee of the board. This example is structured for a board that has the role statement that was quoted in chapter 7.

You may regard the sample QC role statement as being too expansive (or not expansive enough) for your hospital. Clearly the role of board quality committees will vary from hospital to hospital. However, the sample role statement explicitly defines what the QC will do, when it will do it, and the committee's relationship to the board, as well as its relationship to other groups within the hospital.

A role statement is critical in order to distinguish the role of the QC from that of the board, and to facilitate maximum support of the board's oversight of quality. It is also very useful as a tool to evaluate the performance of the QC and to make periodic modifications in the role statement, annual work plan, and structure and composition of the QC to improve its function and support of the board.

Structural Options for a Board Quality Committee

The sample role statement in the previous section implies a particular organizational structure, which is represented by the chart in figure 8-2. The flowchart describes a structure where all groups and activities related to quality report to the board through the QC. This may be an appropriate organizational structure for many hospitals, but it is certainly not the only possible one.

Figure 8-1. Sample Role Statement of the Board Quality Committee

Purpose. The purpose of the Quality Committee of the Board (QC) is to assist the board in oversee-ing and constantly improving the quality of care of this hospital. The QC will assist the board by reviewing and monitoring the following: the information that relates to the quality of care of the hospital, the medical staff credentialing function, the effectiveness of the Quality Assurance (QA) Program and all quality improvement activities, the completeness and effectiveness of the medical staff participation in QA and quality improvement activities, the Risk Management Program, the Infection Control Program, and the Patient Representative Program. The QC will report to the board summary information and conclusions resulting from its monitoring activities as well as recommendations for board action to improve the quality of care, increase the effectiveness of QA and quality improve-ment activities, and minimize the risks of injury to patients and of malpractice losses to the hospital.

Functions. More specifically, the QC will:

1. *Recommend a series of between 12 and 20 quality indicators for regular review by the board and recommend initial threshold levels for those indicators.* Additionally, the QC shall develop and recommend to the board a set of additional quality indicators. Following board approval of the additional quality indicators, the QC shall regularly monitor the indicators and shall bring trends in any of those indicators to the attention of the board when they cross pre-established thresholds or otherwise warrant attention or action by the board. The QC shall also evaluate the effective-ness of the board quality indicators, thresholds, and reporting formats on an annual basis and shall recommend modifications and refinements to them to the board.

2. *Receive from the Medical Executive Committee written recommendations on applications for appoint-ment and reappointment to the medical staff, and privileges delineations.* The QC shall compare the written recommendations of the medical staff to the pre-established level 1 and level 2 criteria for medical staff membership, membership renewal, and privileges delineation. The QC shall then separate the written recommendations of the medical staff into two groups: (1) those where the recommendations are consistent with the criteria profile for each applicant and (2) those where the recommendations are inconsistent with the criteria profile for each applicant or where insuffi-cient information exists to determine consistency of the recommendation to the criteria profile. The QC shall forward all medical staff recommendations from group 1 (recommendations consis-tent with criteria profile) to the full board for action. The QC shall refer all recommendations from group 2 (recommendations inconsistent with criteria profile or with insufficient information) back to the Medical Executive Committee, and shall highlight the discrepancies or areas of insufficient information and request that the Medical Executive Committee review and revise the recommen-dations to make them consistent and complete before resubmitting them to the QC.

3. *Continuously monitor and assess the outcomes and effectiveness of the QA and quality improvement processes of the hospital and of the medical staff.* The QC shall report to the board those areas and departments of the hospital that have the most effective QA activities, as well as those that have the least effective QA activities. The QC shall on an ongoing basis make recommendations to the board for improving the effectiveness of these activities, as well as for improving the quality of care.

4. *Continuously monitor and assess the effectiveness of the hospital's Risk Management Program.* The QC shall provide to the board at least every six months information on the frequency, severity, and causes of patient injuries and adverse patient events; as well as information on the actions taken and the effectiveness of those actions, to reduce the frequency and severity of patient injuries and adverse events. The QC shall monitor the Risk Management Program to verify that a majority of its resources are devoted to the identification and prevention of iatrogenic injuries to patients.

5. *Direct and oversee the annual evaluation of the QA Program and QA Plan.* The QC shall provide the board with the annual evaluation along with recommendations for the improvement of the QA Program and its related activities, and the QA Plan.

6. *Perform the specific tasks and functions that are specified by the board in the annual work plan for the QC.* Additionally, the QC shall perform other specific tasks and duties that are assigned to it by the board.

Figure 8-2. Sample Organizational Chart for a Board with a Quality Committee

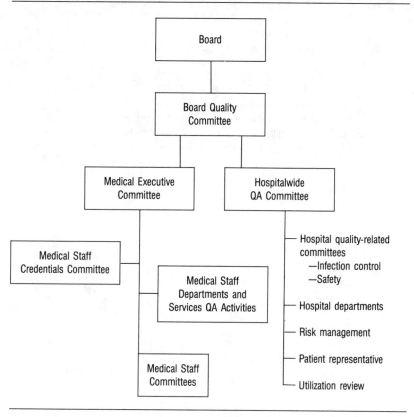

A common issue in organizational structures and information flow relative to a QC involves the medical staff credentialing function and the reporting of medical staff quality assurance activities. In some hospitals the medical staff, for political or other reasons, objects to its credentialing recommendations and other decisions going to a committee of the board, preferring instead that they go directly to the board. In other hospitals, the board wants medical staff recommendations to bypass the QC. Regardless of the political situation, this structure can be a viable one and is fairly common. This type of organizational relationship between the board, the QC, and the medical staff is graphically shown in figure 8-3.

Clearly, the QC represented in figure 8-3 would have a role statement that is different from the one in figure 8-2. The difference in function is that the QC would not address either medical staff credentialing or medical staff quality issues, and the board represented in figure 8-3

Figure 8-3. Sample Organizational Chart for a Board Quality Committee That Does Not Review Medical Staff QA or Credentials Information and Recommendations

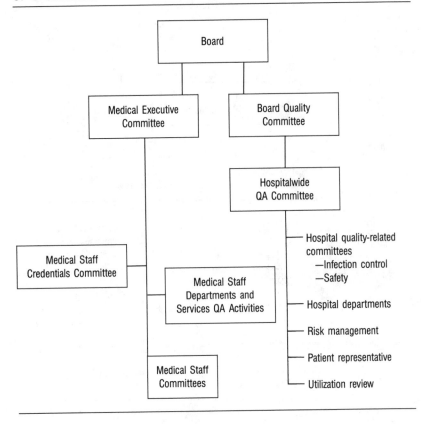

would have to devote its time to consideration of each medical staff credentialing recommendation. For a hospital with a fairly small medical staff, this might not be a problem. For a hospital with a large medical staff, however, this means that the board would be spending quite a bit of its time on medical staff credentialing to perform that function well and appropriately.

The most common problem with the organizational structures described in the previous two paragraphs and in figure 8-3 is the tendency for the board's consideration and oversight of quality activities to become somewhat disjointed. The QC addresses and screens all aspects of quality of care except those that relate to the medical staff, and the medical staff credentialing and QA issues go directly to the board. Clearly the medical staff activities play a significant role in your hospital's quality efforts. So a board in this situation must make certain that it spends time and energy to effectively integrate the quality-related reports from the QC with those of the medical staff to form a true hospitalwide picture of quality. Additionally, this situation can make it difficult for a board to direct quality improvement activities when quality problems or issues cut across organizational lines to involve the medical staff and other parts of the hospital, as they often do.

There are many different organizational structures possible regarding the board, a QC, and quality and its many facets. The important thing for you and your board to bear in mind is that the structure flows from and supports the function. In other words, once you define the role of your QC and its functions, you also will have defined its organizational structure. The function should be defined first, and then the structure created to best support that function.

Composition of a Board Quality Committee

Another important issue that relates to the structure and function of a QC is the composition and the size of the committee. Of course, the composition of the QC will closely relate to the defined role and function of the QC. There are, however, only two basic options to consider regarding the composition of a QC: a committee composed only of board members or a committee composed of trustees, physicians, and hospital management.

Proponents of the first option argue that it is a board committee and thus should be composed entirely of board members. They also make the point that serving on the committee could be a conflict of interest for members of the hospital's medical staff.

Advocates of the second option argue that quality improvement is obtained only through organizationwide commitment and involvement, and that this speaks to the need for a mixed committee. They add that physicians are useful members of a board QC because of their clinical competence and because they can help gain medical staff acceptance of the QC and the board's oversight of quality and the medical staff.

Although your board may have its own perspective on this issue, we advocate the second option. If your board has or establishes a QC, it should be composed of a majority of trustees but should include physicians and management staff. This will provide many benefits to the QC, such as different perspectives and expertise, but it will also pose some challenges. The Hospital Trustees of New York State (1988) point this out:

> The strength of a Board Quality Assurance Committee resides not only in its direct relationship to the Governing Board of the hospital, but in its makeup which . . . blends trustees, administrators, and

physicians. Blending these individuals, however, requires attention to the communications process because the members come from different backgrounds, have different roles to play in the quality assurance process, and sometimes speak different "languages" by virtue of these roles. Physicians can succumb to clinical descriptions which trustees do not comprehend. Administrative staff often have to play a bridging role. . . . The quality assurance professional in these instances has to play a role of interpreter and translator.

The last point is worthy of emphasis. Whether as a member of the QC or as its staff person, your hospital's QA professional should be an integral part of the committee. Further, this individual is the resident expert in quality, quality assurance, and the many related activities in your hospital. As such, the QA professional can be a valuable asset to your board in its quest for quality.

Other Options for Board Oversight of Quality

As mentioned in the beginning of this chapter, there are other alternatives to a QC. In addition, certain structural actions can complement the function of a QC as well as the effectiveness of board oversight of quality.

One of these actions is assigning board members to various committees throughout the hospital that deal with quality. The most appropriate and usual committees for this are the hospitalwide QA committee and the credentials committee of the medical staff. It is appropriate for trustees to be voting members of the hospitalwide QA committee but not so with the credentials committee. For many reasons, some legal and some political, trustee participation in the credentials committee or other committees of the medical staff is most appropriate in the form of ex-officio member without vote, or invited guest.

There are several advantages to having trustees on quality-related committees in the hospital. One major advantage is that it clearly communicates the commitment of the board to quality, medical staff oversight, and related issues. Another is that it allows the board to assess the effectiveness of the function of the various committees by the personal presence of the trustee at the various committees and the subsequent verbal report of the trustee members to the full board, as opposed to the board relying solely on the written reports of the committees themselves.

If your board has a QC, trustee membership on other quality-related committees may help the overall effort but is not critical to it. If your board does not have a QC, however, then trustee membership on quality-related committees is more important to ensuring effective board oversight of the function of those committees and to validating the quality-related information that those committees send to the board.

Boards that do not have QCs must nevertheless ensure that they receive meaningful quality-related information and effectively oversee the quality and medical staff of their hospital. Although it may mean more actual board agenda time spent on the issues of quality and medical staff credentialing, it is not an impossible task. If your board takes this route, try to make certain that it uses the techniques for board oversight of quality outlined in chapter 7 and for oversight of the medical staff credentialing process outlined in chapter 6. Additionally, assigning members of the board to other quality-related committees will help your board discharge its responsibility more effectively.

Although your board does not necessarily need a board-level quality committee and as a whole can effectively oversee the quality of your hospital, you should understand the inherent risks of doing so. For example, your board can become too far removed from the quality assurance, quality improvement, medical staff credentialing, and other activities. Like the hospital boards of the 1950s, your board may come to place more and more trust in the management and medical staff, and rely less on meaningful governance information. This can then lead to the misguided belief that "someone else takes care of quality," and result in an abdication of the board's responsibility. Such abdication will not always happen in the event a board does not have a QC; it is, however, a major risk. The key to avoiding this pitfall is to ensure that your board receives information about quality that is clear, concise, and meaningful—regardless of the board's organizational structure.

Quality and Open Board Meetings

Perhaps the most difficult dilemma that faces some boards regarding quality is the issue of open board meetings. Certain government, state, county, district, and other hospitals are required by law or by their own bylaws to hold board meetings that are open to the public and the press. These boards have trustees who are understandably concerned about discussing sensitive or confidential quality-related issues and then reading about it in the next morning's newspaper. Physicians at these hospitals are also not particularly pleased at the prospect of discussing medical staff credentialing recommendations in a public forum.

Regardless of the difficulties presented by mandatory open board meetings, the boards of these hospitals are still responsible for overseeing quality and medical staff credentialing. How, then, do they do it? Unfortunately, they frequently do not do it well.

There are really very limited alternatives for boards in this situation. The first is to have a quality committee of the board, where a significant majority of the board are members of the QC. The QC considers all the confidential quality and medical staff credentialing information and then makes very terse recommendations to the full board. The full board in turn "rubber stamps" these recommendations.

This solution works wonderfully as long as the *committees* of the board are allowed to meet in closed session. To complicate matters, however, at some hospitals even the committees of the board must meet in open session.

There are only two alternatives for boards in this situation. The first one is that the board concentrates on having very boring meetings so that the press and public stop attending. Then the board addresses quality at those meetings where press and public are absent (don't laugh — some hospital boards deliberately adopt this strategy). For obvious reasons, this is not a particularly viable strategy.

The other alternative is for the board to assign most, if not all, of its members to the quality-related committees of the hospital. These committees then make very terse recommendations to the full board without any accompanying information, and the full board simply "rubber stamps" the recommendations. In any event, open board meetings pose a unique set of problems for a board that is interested in improving its oversight of quality and the medical staff.

Conclusion

Good organizational structure is valuable in supporting good organizational function. As you are well aware, the function of board oversight of quality can be complicated because of the many diverse components of the organization that must be overseen. The complicated functional task of board oversight of quality often manifests in structural difficulties. This in turn gives rise to the temptation to generate structural solutions to what are basically functional problems.

Creating a board quality committee will not in and of itself solve problems in your board's oversight of quality or increase your board's effectiveness in medical staff credentialing decisions. Without careful thought and planning, structural changes can easily create more problems as well as exacerbate existing ones.

The structural aspects of your board's involvement in quality should be created for the express purpose of supporting explicitly defined roles and functions. In this way the structure of a quality committee of your board, or trustee membership on quality-related committees of the hospital, can truly support and facilitate your board's effective involvement in and oversight of quality in your hospital.

References

Orlikoff, J. E. *Quality from the Top: Working with Hospital Governing Boards to Assure Quality Care—A Guide for Quality Assurance Professionals.* Chicago: Pluribus Press, 1990.

Hospital Trustees of New York State. *The Model Hospital Board Quality Assurance Project: A Study of Trustee Involvement in Quality Assurance Management.* Albany, NY: Hospital Association of New York State, 1988.

New Approaches in Quality: Continuous Quality Improvement

Introduction

Health care history books may well label the 1990s the beginning of the "quality era" in health care delivery. Today, more and more hospitals are moving away from a primary emphasis on cost control toward a focus on broader strategies that can help ensure survival and success for the long term. As was mentioned earlier, many of these institutions are turning toward improving the quality of the health care services they deliver as a way to become the provider of choice in their communities today and into the future.

As a hospital trustee, you most likely wear several hats in your community. Like many trustees, you may also work in or run a business or community organization. You know from experience that organizations that deliver high-quality products and services are more likely to grow and prosper than those that do not. Just like American businesses and industry, many hospitals are beginning to realize that consistent delivery of a quality product or service builds patient loyalty and employee morale and actually improves productivity and lowers cost over the long run.

The quest for quality in health care today is occurring on several fronts. Some hospitals are finding success in expanding and strengthening their traditional quality assurance programs. These efforts, reviewed in depth in earlier chapters, often include responding more to patient satisfaction surveys or feedback from patient representatives, fostering greater physician involvement in quality assurance activities, focusing more on the outcome of care delivery as a primary indicator of quality, or prospectively building quality into programs and services before they are launched. Whereas some experts suggest that these activities make important contributions to improving quality, others fear they may stop short of the type of organizationwide commitment to quality that is necessary to support ongoing, long-term improvement.

This chapter will discuss a major new theory and initiative in the search for quality in health care—the concept of Continuous Quality Improvement (CQI), also referred to as Total Quality Management (TQM). Hailed as a "substantive alternative to traditional methods of quality assurance" (O'Leary, 1990, p. 2), CQI is becoming a way of life for many providers.

Continuous Quality Improvement

Continuous quality improvement is a customer-focused, quality-driven philosophy and process that relies on each member of an organization to build quality into every step of service development and delivery. Advocates of CQI theory contrast it to the "theory of bad apples," which they say has characterized traditional industrial and hospital quality assurance efforts.

The bad apple theory relies heavily on inspection methods and processes to identify those responsible for errors or problems. Continuous quality improvement theory, on the other hand, discards the witch-hunt approach to improving quality in favor of seeking to involve everyone in continuously examining the systems and processes they use to accomplish their work. The goal of this ongoing examination is to identify problems and correct them so that the system improves. In the processes of creating and delivering products or services, CQI focuses on reducing errors, waste, and rework, thereby ultimately improving quality.

Organizations that adopt and implement CQI often undergo nothing less than a major transformation in the ways they think about and accomplish their work. And those that have been most successful have developed and sustained their quality vision and commitment at the top. As Brent James of Intermountain Healthcare (1990, p. 26) suggests: "High quality depends primarily on good leadership. . . . It begins in the boardroom . . . and requires a long-term, hands-on commitment from the top leaders in an organization."

As a member of your hospital's governing board you will have the opportunity to help define, shape, and support your hospital's commitment to quality. The following discussion shows how CQI is changing the way many hospitals operate. It also will help you, as a governing board member, understand the role you can play in fostering and sustaining a long-term vision for quality in your hospital.

History and Development

Although the concept of CQI was developed more than 60 years ago, it was not until the late 1970s that it began to be embraced and applied by U.S. industries. Ironically, although CQI theory was developed by American statisticians, it was first tested and applied in post–World War II Japan (Orlikoff and Snow, 1984, pp. 2–5).

Prior to World War II, Japanese industrial development lagged significantly behind that of Western industrialized nations. At that time, Japanese products had a worldwide reputation for consistently poor quality. "Made in Japan" was synonymous with cheap, short-lived products that often broke or malfunctioned soon after they were purchased. Pre–World War II Japanese industry had focused on carving out a small niche in world markets by using cheap labor to produce cheap products and emphasizing quantity over quality.

After World War II, the United States focused on helping Japan achieve a strong economic recovery. Because Japan's natural resources were extremely limited, the nation adopted a strategy of providing quality products as the best way to compete more effectively in world markets. General Douglas MacArthur, who commanded the U.S. occupation forces in Japan, and the Japanese industrialists he assigned to lead the nation's economic recovery all realized that Japan's greatest natural resource was its people. This realization, coupled with a focus on quality to drive industrial expansion, set the stage for the application of CQI.

To help provide the Japanese with tools to facilitate the nation's economic recovery, MacArthur contacted W. Edwards Deming, Ph.D., an American statistician who had developed statistical and management methods to improve product quality and worker productivity. Deming's ideas and techniques had not sparked the interest of U.S. companies, but at the request of the Japanese he went to Japan to teach his methods.

Deming taught the Japanese statistical techniques to control and therefore improve product quality. He also advocated the idea that quality cannot be inspected into a product but must be built in at every step of production. Deming's statistical control methods and his concepts of building quality into products along the way formed the basics of Japan's developing science of quality control.

It was not until the early 1950s that the Japanese concept of quality control moved beyond the realm of scientists and engineers and into the hands of production supervisors and workers. This expansion was facilitated by Joseph M. Juran, another American interested in improving quality and productivity. Juran's lectures to Japanese industrial leaders convinced them that quality was everyone's responsibility. The idea of involving all employees in achieving total quality control became a national goal for Japan.

Out of this concept that everyone should participate in achieving quality grew the development of *quality control circles*—groups of workers from the same or similar work areas trained to apply the techniques of quality control to identify and solve problems in their work processes. Although quality control circles were first started as a way to teach workers the principles of quality control, they soon became the mechanism used to actually implement quality control techniques and achieve quality improvement.

It was not until the late 1960s that the idea of quality control circles came to the United States. In the mid- to late 1970s they were first adopted by U.S. industries, where they were renamed *quality circles* to avoid the negative connotations and limited scope implied by the word *control*.

In the early 1980s, quality circles moved beyond product-focused industries and began to be adopted by service-oriented industries, including hospitals. However, what both product and service industries discovered was that using quality circles alone does not necessarily sustain and improve quality over time. What is needed is a top-down vision of and commitment to quality as the number one organizational goal. Those organizations that have made quality the primary, strategic thrust have introduced and applied the CQI principles and techniques first developed by Deming, Juran, and the Japanese throughout their organizations. They also have taken to heart and applied the philosophy of CQI—a total commitment to involving everyone in continuously seeking to improve quality over the long term. These organizations have found that establishing and sustaining a culture for quality is the key to continued quality improvement. Furthermore, they have learned that the commitment to such a culture begins in the boardroom.

In the late 1980s, interest accelerated in applying CQI techniques in hospitals. Applications have occurred in large multihospital systems such as the Health Care Corporation of America, managed care environments such as the Harvard Community Health Plan, and in freestanding community hospitals as well. By the mid-1990s the Joint Commission on Accreditation of Healthcare Organizations, which has applied CQI techniques internally, is expected to publish quality standards for hospitals based on CQI principles. In addition, large corporate purchasers of health care are beginning to require that hospitals that provide health care to their employees must practice CQI.

As a board member, you may be wondering just what CQI is all about and whether or not it might make sense for your hospital. The rest of this chapter is devoted to describing CQI and helping you evaluate its potential for your institution. The next section of this chapter describes the CQI philosophy in more detail. Understanding the principles on which CQI is based can help you better understand the important role board members play in paving the way for CQI in their hospitals.

The CQI Philosophy

At this point you might be thinking, with some degree of frustration, "Why have I just read an entire book on my role in assuring quality when the field may be abandoning the traditional quality assurance approach in favor of continuous quality improvement?" Be assured that your efforts to understand quality assurance have not been in vain. In fact, comparing and contrasting QA and CQI may help you better see how elements of both can be combined into a more effective and enduring way to achieve real, shortand long-term improvements in your hospital's quality of care.

Dennis O'Leary, president of the Joint Commission (1990, p. 2), has described CQI as a step beyond QA:

Both the differences and similarities between CQI and QA are meaningful. In simple terms, CQI is built from the foundation of the positive aspects of QA but seeks to redirect the focus of organizational attention on quality of care issues. . . .

O'Leary points out that the terms *QA* and *CQI* convey different meanings. *Quality assurance,* he says, has been traditionally viewed as a blame-finding, compartmentalized activity focused on generating specific requirements for individual departments in the hospital, often with the goal of meeting external regulations or standards. He stated:

In retrospect, the word "assurance" was an unfortunate semantic selection. Quality of course could never be assured, it could only be improved. . . . Meanwhile, the emphasis of QA on identifying "problems" and "outliers" took its toll inside organizations. Not surprisingly, it was (and is) difficult for a negatively oriented process to capture the support and imagination of health care professionals.

As O'Leary and others who have written about CQI point out, CQI is based on a different philosophy and set of assumptions. What Deming, Juran, and others discovered while studying the sources of quality problems was that the problems, and therefore the opportunities to solve them, were part of the systems and processes used to create products. Rarely were they attributable to the lack of will, skill, or intention of individual workers. Even when people were causing defects, the root of the problem most often could be traced to poor job design, leadership failure, or unclear purpose.

Therefore, these quality researchers discovered, it becomes more productive to study the systems used to produce a product or service and correct flaws in these systems as the way to improve quality, rather than looking to blame individuals for quality problems. This approach recognizes the humanity and complexity of organizations and seeks to achieve improvement through positive motivation and group effort rather than by the spread of fear and disaffection engendered by a disciplinary approach.

The core of CQI and perhaps its most basic principle is that systems can always be improved. Organizations that use CQI make the continuous search for improvement in the processes used to create products and services a way of life. As Donald Berwick, M.D., of the Harvard Community Health Plan (1989, p. 54), suggests:

> The focus is on continuous improvement throughout the organization through constant effort to reduce waste, rework, and complexity. When one is clear and constant in one's purpose, where fear does not control the atmosphere . . . when learning is guided by accurate information and sound rules of inference, when suppliers of services remain in dialogue with those who depend on them and when the hearts and talents of all workers are enlisted in the pursuit of better ways, the potential for improvement in quality is nearly boundless.

Seeking quality improvement through the study of work systems and processes, focusing on group rather than individual effort, and making the search for quality a continuous, organizationwide activity are basic principles of the CQI philosophy. But CQI is more than a philosophy or vision. It employs specific tools, techniques, and approaches that can be used to systematically achieve quality improvement.

The next section of this chapter discusses the activities, tools and techniques used in practicing CQI, beginning with the role of the governing board and other hospital leaders in establishing a culture for quality within which CQI can succeed.

The CQI Process

Most organizations that have implemented CQI say that long-term success depends on the support and involvement of the organization's leaders. The CQI process does not take root or show results overnight. Organizations implementing CQI realistically can expect a five-year time line from planning and start-up through initial results. That is why organizations generally do not take on a commitment to CQI lightly.

In those organizations that systematically adopt CQI, many of the early months of the process are devoted to educating the organization's leadership about CQI—its definition, principles and practices, and implications for change. Once a common understanding of CQI is reached at the top, the leadership group then devotes its time and energy to determining whether CQI is right for the organization. If the leaders agree to adopt CQI, then they must define what CQI means for the organization and appropriately express that definition in and outside the organization.

Development of a quality mission statement that sets forth the organization's quality vision is the first responsibility that the hospital board undertakes to implement CQI. According to James (1990, p. 26), a quality mission statement should specify:

- Constancy of purpose
- Dedication to continuous improvement
- Focus on the customer (broadly defined as patients, payers, physicians, and employees)
- Understanding of the product or service
- Measurement systems to evaluate quality

Establishing a context within which CQI can develop—creating a culture for quality—can't be delegated. As a board member it is important for you to understand that once the board makes the decision to adopt CQI, its work has just begun. The organization's leaders must spearhead and guide the transformation to ensure long-lasting success.

Many organizations begin to address the specifics of CQI implementation by devising a short-term strategic plan that maps out the first year or two of development. In other words, this plan lays the groundwork for getting started. It should address:

- Where the CQI process might first be successfully tried in the organization
- What resources—financial and human—will be needed to train employees, establish CQI projects, and lend support and guidance to organizational managers, supervisors, and project teams
- How logistics and organizationwide communication and implementation will be coordinated (Scholtes, 1988, p. 1–15)

As a board member, your role not only includes establishing the quality mission and becoming an agent for change by communicating the mission, but also overseeing development of the CQI strategic plan, both the short-term plan described above and a longer-term plan as well. You and the members of your board also will vote to allocate the resources necessary to implement CQI and monitor the implementation of the strategic plan to ensure that the organization stays on course and continues to fulfill its commitment to quality.

The Basics of Continuous Quality Improvement

To implement CQI, the organization needs to understand the underlying philosophy of quality improvement as well as the specific tools, techniques, and approaches that can be used to achieve it. As a board member, familiarity with some CQI basics can help you understand how the CQI process works and can better help you evaluate how effective it might be in your hospital.

The CQI philosophy has been summarized by Dr. Deming in what have become widely known as Deming's 14 points and 7 deadly diseases (see figures 9-1 and 9-2). These ideas are often discussed for several hours during CQI training sessions so that everyone can appreciate their meaning and significance and arrive at a common understanding of what CQI is all about.

Approaches to teaching the CQI process vary, some focusing on classroom learning followed by implementation and others focusing on learning by doing. Although approaches may differ, all emphasize common elements essential to CQI effectiveness. Key elements or aspects of the CQI process are described in the following paragraphs (Scholtes, 1988, pp. 2-2 to 2-46).

Determining Processes and Systems

Continuous quality improvement stresses viewing the work of an organization as series of steps, which group into processes, which then group

Figure 9-1. Deming's 14 Points for Continuous Quality Improvement

1. Create constancy of purpose.

2. Adopt a new philosophy.

3. Cease dependence on inspection to achieve quality.

4. End the practice of awarding business on price tag alone. Instead, minimize total cost.

5. Improve constantly and forever the system of production and service.

6. Institute training on the job.

7. Institute leadership.

8. Drive out fear.

9. Break down barriers between departments.

10. Eliminate slogans, exhortations, and targets for the work force asking for zero defects and new levels of productivity.

11. Eliminate quotas for the work force and management by numerical goals.

12. Remove barriers that rob workers and management of their right to pride of workmanship.

13. Institute a vigorous program of education and self-improvement.

14. Put everyone in the company to work to accomplish the transformation.

Figure 9-2. The Seven Deadly Diseases Inhibiting Quality Improvement

1. Lack of constancy of purpose to plan products and services that will help keep the company in business and provide jobs.

2. Emphasis on short-term profits.

3. Use of performance reviews and management by objective.

4. Job hopping.

5. Use of visible performance data for management only, with no consideration of the unknown or unknowable.

6. Excessive medical costs.

7. Excessive liability costs.

into systems. The delivery of obstetrical care, for example, is a system involving a number of interrelated processes, such as prenatal care, delivery of the child, and postpartum care. Each of these processes in turn breaks down into a series of related steps. Even though the idea of breaking down the work of the organization into systems, processes, and steps may sound simple and straightforward, thinking in these terms is one of the most profound changes that occurs in the transformation to CQI. Many new insights often are gained when participants see how tasks are related and how the work they perform fits into a broader whole. Focusing on processes helps people think about how their work actually gets accomplished and is the basis for understanding how improvements can be made.

Understanding Customers and Suppliers

Understanding what customers and suppliers need and desire in a product or service is the basis for understanding what quality means. However, CQI defines customers and suppliers differently than we typically think of them. *Suppliers* are the people or organizations who come before the process identified for study; *customers* are those who follow the process and use the product or service it produces. Therefore, at the most basic level, each worker is a customer of preceding workers and a supplier to the workers who next receive the product.

Achieving Quality

"Quality begins with the customer" is a popular saying in CQI. Only customers, the people who receive your work, can tell you what they want in a product and how they want to receive it. Therefore, to achieve quality the organization must build quality into every step of every process by working with internal and external customers to identify their needs and collaborating with internal and external suppliers to fulfill them. It is important, however, to remember Deming's concept that the responsibility for quality rests at the top of the organization. Only the organization's leaders, including you and the members of your board, can define quality, establish the organization's commitment to it, and bring your power and influence to bear in supporting employees to create and deliver quality products and services to customers.

Maximizing Teamwork

The biggest quality gains most frequently result from teams of workers pooling their knowledge and skills to understand processes and how to improve them. This concept of teams and teamwork is the basis of quality circles discussed earlier. Teams can best tackle complex problems and come up with useful solutions, while supporting each other along the way. The CQI process involves use of a number of group process techniques to explore ideas or make decisions. These can include:

- *Brainstorming.* A process to generate a wide range of ideas or options
- *Multivoting.* A series of votes to pare down a long list of items to a manageable number
- *Nominal group technique.* A structured approach to generate ideas and then narrow them down to key priorities

Utilizing a Scientific Approach

A scientific approach is the core of the quality improvement methodology and provides a systematic way for teams to tackle problems. The scientific approach need not be complex. It involves making decisions by examining data, not on hunches; looking for root causes of problems, not symptoms; and seeking enduring solutions, not Band-Aids or quick fixes. Several tools can assist a team to understand where problems lie and therefore where quality might be improved. A list of common scientific tools and their uses appears in figure 9-3. Examples of how some of these tools might be applied appear in figures 9-4 and 9-5.

Reducing Complexity

Even if root causes are not immediately apparent, project teams often can discover the complexity that evolved to compensate for a given problem. *Complexity* refers to anything that makes a process more complicated without adding any value to the product or service. Four types

of complexity often exist: errors or defects, breakdowns and delays, ineffi-
ciencies, and variation. The last of these, variation, is a major problem
that makes processes less reliable. Eliminating variation as much as
appropriately possible to increase uniformity in output is a goal of CQI.
In other words, finding the simplest and most effective way of doing

---

Figure 9-3.   Common Scientific Tools and Their Uses for Continuous Quality Improvement

Flowchart: A step-by-step picture that can be used to plan the phases of a project or depict a process being studied.

Cause-and-effect diagram: Also known as a fishbone diagram; used to help map out factors thought to affect a problem or outcome.

Scatter diagram: A point plot that shows the possible relationship between two process characteristics.

Checksheet: Used in data collection to record sample observations to begin to detect patterns.

Pareto chart: A bar graph constructed in descending order of priority, where the height of the bar shows the relative importance of the problem.

Histogram: Displays the distribution of data via a bar graph showing the number of units in each category.

Run chart: Plots observation points over time to show trends.

Figure 9-4.   Sample Pareto Chart for Identifying Opportunities for Quality Improvement

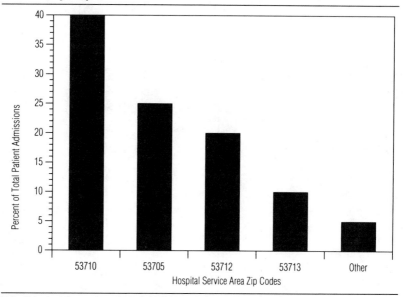

Note: This chart shows a hypothetical distribution of a hospital's patient population throughout its service area, noting levels of concentration by ZIP code.

Figure 9-5. Sample Cause-and-Effect Diagram for Identifying Opportunities for Quality Improvement

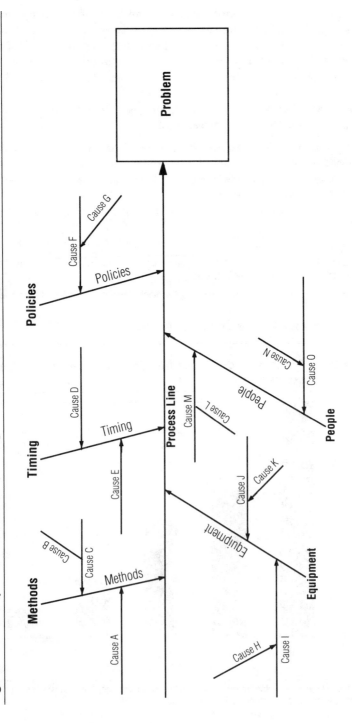

Note: This cause-and-effect, or fishbone, diagram shows various causes that contribute to a problem. For example, causes A, B, and C contribute to a composite of all related causes in the methods category contributing to the larger problem.

something and then consistently doing it that way helps improve quality and lower costs.

Running Statistically Designed Experiments

Statistically designed experiments use a variety of efficient, systematic, and flexible methods that allow several variables to be tested in a single experiment. These experiments have several uses, such as helping to determine optimal operating procedures or conditions for a program or service, or helping to smooth the transition from pilot project to full-scale operation. For example, a quality improvement team in your hospital's central supply area might discover that supplies were not really available for distribution as needed throughout the hospital. The team might test a number of alternative methods for shelving supplies to determine which variables (providing quick access to the most frequently requested items, positioning items to easily determine when stock is low, and so forth) were most important to ensure ongoing availability of needed supplies.

With practice, the methods employed in running statistically designed experiments are not difficult to use. However, these methods are usually learned under the guidance of someone experienced in running designed experiments.

Implementing a CQI Project

Once participants understand the elements and tools of the CQI process, they can begin to select and implement quality improvement projects. The steps involved in implementing a CQI project are depicted in figure 9-6. The continuous examination of work systems and processes using the steps, tools, and techniques described in the previous paragraphs to identify and solve problems is the essence of CQI. Continuous quality improvement is therefore an ongoing process that is an end in itself.

CQI Implementation Issues

Hospitals that decide to adopt CQI in earnest will be changing their way of life; such a commitment cannot and should not be made lightly. Although many hospitals already have found success in applying CQI, they had to overcome some hurdles along the way. Being aware of issues that can affect the successful implementation of CQI in health care settings will help you determine whether CQI is right for your hospital (Fainter, 1989).

Figure 9-6. Quality Project Milestones

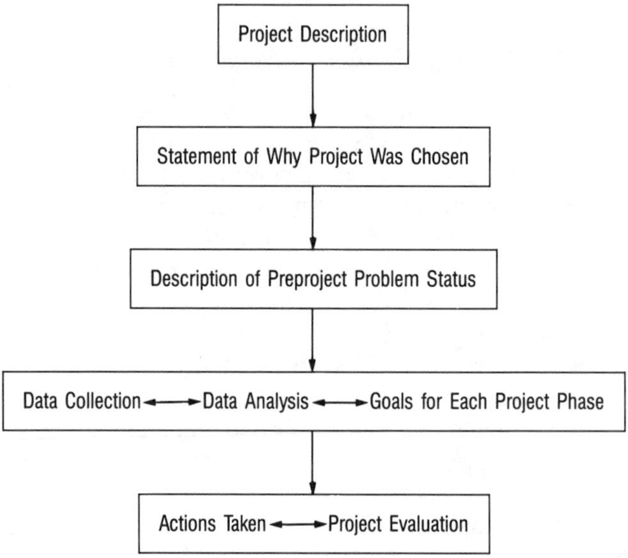

```
                    ┌─────────────────────────┐
                    │    Project Description   │
                    └─────────────────────────┘
                                 │
                                 ▼
          ┌──────────────────────────────────────┐
          │  Statement of Why Project Was Chosen  │
          └──────────────────────────────────────┘
                                 │
                                 ▼
        ┌───────────────────────────────────────────┐
        │  Description of Preproject Problem Status  │
        └───────────────────────────────────────────┘
                                 │
                                 ▼
  ┌────────────────────────────────────────────────────────────┐
  │ Data Collection ◄──► Data Analysis ◄──► Goals for Each Project Phase │
  └────────────────────────────────────────────────────────────┘
                                 │
                                 ▼
          ┌──────────────────────────────────────┐
          │  Actions Taken ◄──► Project Evaluation │
          └──────────────────────────────────────┘
```

A Participative Philosophy and Process

Continuous quality improvement is based on the notion that everyone works together to achieve quality improvement. In most organizations, this means that the CQI process will increase employee involvement in decision making. If a hospital's management or medical staff does not want to share decision making with employees, CQI probably will never work. This point bears repeating. Resistance to a participative management style is often the single biggest reason why CQI is never introduced or never gets off the ground.

Knowing the Customer

Who are our customers? How do they define quality? What do they want in our products and services? Knowing the answers to these questions is central to achieving quality improvement in CQI. Organizations that tackle these questions prior to CQI implementation understand that quality really does begin with the customer.

Differences between Health Care and Other Industries

Many who are skeptical of CQI question whether statistical process control techniques and applications developed in industrial settings are right for service-oriented industries. "After all," they say, "hospitals don't make widgets—they treat patients."

This discomfort stems from a number of factors. The delivery of health care is a complex, often emotionally charged process based on hundreds of individual interactions between providers and patients. This complexity and focus on individuality rather than commonality have caused some to question the applicability and appropriateness of a process that seeks to diminish variation to achieve more uniform output. A traditional reliance on problem solving rather than process improvement, a history of departmentalized quality assurance rather than organizationwide quality improvement, a relatively recent imperative in health care to link cost and quality, and a long history of mixing art and science in the practice of medicine also breed resistance to applying CQI in hospitals. Whereas several hospitals and health care systems have found that CQI can work—that there are common steps in the process of correctly admitting a patient, dispensing medication, or conducting hundreds of other health care delivery processes—many within the health care industry remain skeptical.

The Physician's Role

Perhaps one of the greatest challenges to introducing CQI in hospitals is gaining the acceptance and participation of physicians. If you think about physicians' traditional role in the health care system, it's not difficult to understand why they are likely to have a negative reaction to CQI. Physicians have historically operated independently and are used to having power and control in the health care setting. They are used to participating in processes like peer review that equate quality improvement with individual case review rather than the study of care delivery processes in which the physician's role is only a part. Because many CQI techniques come out of the theory of group process and teamwork, physicians may be largely unfamiliar with them. And, given that physicians are currently beleaguered by a host of problems—diminishing power and respect in the health care system, decreasing income, and increasing loss of professional freedom, to name a few—they are likely to be suspicious of a process that requires a lot of their time and that seems to have little to do with their primary focus on individual patient care (Merry, 1990, pp. 101–103).

On the other hand, physicians who have tried CQI techniques report that they greatly improve their own problem-solving and quality improvement capabilities. Physicians who have practiced CQI also point out that physicians create and use dozens of processes both in care delivery and in running their practices. Scheduling patients, issuing bills, prescribing medication, or giving a patient instructions are just a few of the hundreds of processes that exist in the practice of medicine and that can be improved by the use of systematic techniques (Berwick, 1989, p. 55). Some physicians using CQI maintain that physicians will find quality improvement tools and techniques intuitively appealing because they are scientifically based (Schlosser, 1989).

The key to effectively involving physicians in CQI lies in helping them understand the CQI payoff—how CQI can empower them to be active, effective participants in quality improvement in the hospital and in their individual practices. According to CQI supporters, controlling unnecessary and harmful variation in the delivery of care can help physicians make inroads toward greater economic stability, gain a greater sense of participation and influence in the hospital's future development and success, maintain sufficient clinical freedom to deal with the uncertainties of patient care, and perhaps restore a lost sense of the social value and respect associated with the physician's work (Merry, 1990, p. 104). Therefore, CQI becomes the key ingredient in a win-win strategy for physicians and all participants in the CQI process.

How CQI Relates to Quality Assurance

"If we adopt CQI," you might ask, "what happens to our quality assurance program?" This chapter has compared and contrasted CQI and QA and discussed how CQI has grown out of the positive aspects of QA. It also has demonstrated that CQI is a data-based process that relies on the collection and interpretation of quality-related information—much of which already exists in the hospital. The hospital's quality assurance program can be the source for much of the data needed by CQI project teams to identify and solve problems. Hospitals that adopt CQI may want to designate their quality assurance program to be a central source for collection of a variety of quality-related data—clinical and risk management data, employee and patient feedback, and the like. The difference is that the CQI process relies on teams of workers who have identified problems to integrate and interpret these data and apply them within and across work areas as necessary to improve quality organizationwide.

Reasonable Expectations for Quality Improvement

Organizations committed to CQI understand that resource allocation, education, training, testing, learning from mistakes—taking the time to get it right—all precede achievement of measurable, sustainable results. This is not to say that CQI pilot successes cannot help gain commitment for CQI throughout your hospital or that early projects are never successful. The point is that education is an ongoing process and that seeking broad-based results before commitment will likely contribute to the failure of CQI in your hospital. That's why organizations that truly make the commitment seek first to understand CQI, debate its merits, try to determine what obstacles may exist and whether they can be overcome to help ensure successful adoption of CQI over the long term. Much of this initial education, debate, soul-searching, and analysis takes place among the organization's leaders. The next section of this chapter is designed to help you and the members of your board assess whether CQI will work in your hospital.

Is Your Hospital Ready for CQI?

Now that you understand the CQI philosophy and process and some of the common issues and concerns affecting successful CQI implementation, you and your board can evaluate whether your hospital is ready for CQI. The following list of questions can help you pinpoint your organizational strengths and weaknesses related to CQI readiness and help you determine the steps that would need to be taken to pave the way for CQI.

- *CQI validity for hospitals:* Do we believe that CQI can be effectively applied to the delivery of health care? What has been the experience of other hospitals? Is this the right solution for us at this time?
- *History of organizational acceptance of change:* What have been management, employee, and physician attitudes toward other new programs that have been implemented—employee morale, hospital image, or flex-time programs, for example? Where has resistance traditionally been most frequent and strong?
- *Current organizational status and climate:* Is our hospital financially healthy? Are we growing, remaining static, or declining? What about our competitors? How would we characterize current employee morale and attitudes? What about employee–management–physician relationships? If we implement CQI now, can we sustain it over the long term?
- *Management acceptance:* Does our hospital's top management understand CQI, and will they likely support and be motivated to implement it? Will our middle managers, often the key to effective implementation, support and sustain CQI, or will they view it as another executive directive or fad?
- *Physician acceptance:* How will our physicians view CQI? Are they likely to oppose it or support it over the long term?
- *Time and resources:* Do we have the time and the human and financial resources to educate and train everyone in CQI? Do we have

enough internal resources to do the job, or do we need to acquire them or obtain outside support?

- *Liability issues:* If CQI involves developing stronger relationships with others outside the hospital who help us deliver our services, do we face any potential confidentiality problems or other liability issues?

- *Union acceptance:* If our hospital is unionized, do we face any contract, work rule, or other limitations that would hinder effective CQI implementation?

- *External factors:* Will our current suppliers be likely to participate successfully with us in a CQI environment, or will we need to develop new relationships? Can we implement CQI and still meet other regulatory, legal, and legislative requirements? What advantages or disadvantages might CQI present for our hospital's competitive position? How will our community react?

Although this set of questions is not meant to be all-inclusive, it gives you and your board a starting point for assessing whether your hospital can take on CQI and make it work. If you determine that the majority of these issues are not problems for your hospital or that they are problems that can be successfully resolved, then you are ready to determine your commitment to CQI and the steps that should be taken to make CQI a way of life for your hospital.

Conclusion

This chapter has discussed a major new milestone in the quest for quality in health care, the philosophy and process of continuous quality improvement. It has traced the origin of the CQI concept and explained the underlying principles, tools, and techniques that make up CQI. Major issues and concerns that may hinder CQI implementation were discussed, as well as an approach you and you board might use to assess whether your hospital is ready for CQI.

Continuous quality improvement focuses an organization on one primary goal: long-term, ongoing dedication to continually improving quality. As we hope this chapter has convinced you, CQI represents nothing less than a major transformation for most organizations. Its success relies on a degree of organizational readiness, outlined above, and particularly, acceptance of participative management at all levels. For these reasons, CQI may not be right for some hospitals, at least not until they are motivated and ready to accept it.

As a member of your hospital's governing board, you will likely hear more about CQI and may soon be involved in deliberations about whether it is the right approach for your hospital. Time will tell whether CQI will be perceived as a fad or a foundation for the future in health care. The challenge for you and your governing board is to understand CQI and its likely impact well enough to make that call for your hospital.

References

Berwick, D. M. Sounding board: continuous improvement as an ideal in health care. *New England Journal of Medicine* 320(1):53–56, Jan. 5, 1989.

Fainter, J. Hospital cultural barriers to quality improvement. Presentation at the Joint Commission on Accreditation of Healthcare Organization's National Forum on Health Care Quality Improvement, Rosemont, IL, Nov. 14–17, 1989.

James, B. C. Implementing continuous quality improvement. *Trustee* 43(4):16–17, 26, Apr. 1990.

Merry, M. Total quality management for physicians: translating the new paradigm. *Quality Review Bulletin* 16(3):101–5, Mar. 1990.

O'Leary, D. S. CQI—a step beyond QA. *Joint Commission Perspectives* 10(2):2–3, Mar./Apr. 1990.

Orlikoff, J. E., and Snow, A. *Assessing Quality Circles in Health Care Settings.* Chicago: American Hospital Publishing, 1984.

Schlosser, J. Quality improvement in health care: why it will work and how to involve physicians. *The Quality Letter for Healthcare Leaders* 1(2):10–12, Sept. 1989.

Scholtes, P. R. *The Team Handbook: How to Use Teams to Improve Quality.* Madison, WI: Joiner Associates, 1988.

Chapter 10

Conclusion

Just as the costs of health care eclipsed all other health issues in the 1980s, quality is emerging as an equally dominant and possibly more complex theme of the 1990s and beyond. The cost pressures of the 1980s have evolved into the pressures for your hospital to provide quality care in an environment of diminishing resources. These pressures are compounded by increasing regulatory and public scrutiny of your hospital's quality of care.

As a result, you and your board have probably been hearing a lot about quality recently, and you will continue to hear a lot about quality in the coming years. You will feel external pressure to address and improve quality in your hospital, and you will naturally feel compelled to make certain that your hospital addresses and responds to these external pressures and regulations. Before your board and hospital simply react and respond to these external pressures, you should recognize and accept a simple truth: *Quality comes from within.*

Your hospital can gear up to meet whatever external regulations and requirements come down the pike. Compliance with these regulations and requirements might even result in improvements in your hospital's quality of care. You and your board must understand, however, that a true quest for quality and continuous improvements in quality cannot be externally regulated or mandated; it must be internally motivated.

The internal organizational commitment to and motivation for quality is the foundation that supports and nurtures your hospital's culture for quality. It comes from the conscience of your hospital, from the critical questioner and overseer of your hospital, from the ultimate authority of your hospital. It comes from your board.

The quality of care that your hospital provides begins and ends with your board. Effective board involvement in and oversight of your hospital's quest for quality hinges on two critical components: meaningful commitment to quality, and meaningful information about quality and effective governance response to that information.

A Meaningful Commitment to Quality

Yes, your board has the ultimate responsibility for quality in your hospital. That is easy to say but difficult for an entire board to truly understand. Yet it is necessary for your entire board to understand and accept why it is responsible for quality in order to develop a sincere commitment to quality and the quest to continuously improve it.

Thus your board must take steps to nurture this understanding through board education and discussion until every board member understands and accepts this most important of all board responsibilities. Then your board must make certain that this understanding and commitment is perpetuated via strong orientation programs for new trustees and refresher sessions for experienced board members. Your board's commitment to and performance in overseeing and improving quality should be routinely evaluated and improved as a major component of your regular board self-evaluations. Like quality itself, your board's commitment to and effective oversight of quality can always be improved.

Next, the commitment of your board to the quest for quality must become the base to nurture a true organizational commitment to quality, a culture for quality. This will be a multifaceted process. It will involve the relationship between the board and the hospital chief executive officer as your board communicates its passion for quality to the CEO. The commitment of the board to quality must be more than words to the CEO and management staff. It must take the form of specific CEO and management performance objectives, resource allocations, long-term strategic planning, the performance of prospective quality assurance by the board on major decisions that will impact the quality of care, and continuing board interest and emphasis on quality.

The commitment and resolve of the board must also be communicated to and shared with the medical staff of the hospital. They must be made to understand why quality and its improvement are integral to the very fabric and future of the organization. They must understand that the board is sincere in its commitment and dedication to quality, that this is not just a passing fad but a persistent passion. The methods and techniques for measuring and improving quality will change, but the motivation for and commitment to quality remain constant.

The motivation and commitment of your board to quality must also be communicated to all hospital staff and employees. They, as well as management and medical staff, must realize and accept that quality is their responsibility, that it is everyone's responsibility throughout the organization.

This development of a culture for quality will not come easily or quickly, but it must nevertheless come; and it will come only from your board. Your board must develop a passion for quality and nurture the flames of this passion until they grow and consume and drive your entire hospital.

Meaningful Governance Information about Quality

The second component of effective board oversight of and improvements in quality is meaningful governance information about quality. Your board must make certain that it regularly receives clear, concise governance information about your hospital's quality and the activities to measure and improve it. This information should facilitate action by your board that results in improvements in quality, resolution of problems, and an advancement of the culture of quality throughout your hospital.

A Final Question

This book has attempted to make you more comfortable with the issue of quality, with the board's responsibility for it, and with how your board can and must actively influence and oversee your hospital's quality of care. Quality and your board's role in it should be less of a mystery to you now.

Because true quality is not a goal but rather a journey or quest, this book also has attempted to guide you on that quest. In doing so it began with a question to stimulate your thinking and begin your journey in quality. It is a question you should always ask yourself to keep moving forward in your quest for quality, and so this book will conclude where it began.

Does your hospital deliver high-quality care to its patients?

37.20

American Hospital Publishing, Inc.
737 North Michigan Avenue
Chicago, Illinois 60611

Catalog no. 196126

ISBN 1-55648-061